THE HEALTHY BRAIN TOOLBOX

Neurologist-Proven Strategies
to Prevent Memory Loss and
Protect Your Aging Brain

By Ken Sharlin, MD, MPH, IFMCP

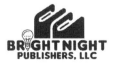

Bright Night Publishers, LLC

First Edition: May 2018

ISBN (Print): 978-1-7320770-1-0
ISBN (ePUB): 978-1-7320770-2-7
ISBN (MOBI): 978-1-7320770-0-3

Interior design by booknook.biz

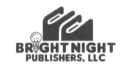

Bright Night Publishers, LLC
5528 N. Farmer Branch Rd.
Ozark, MO 65721

Disclaimer

Neither the publisher nor the author is engaged in rendering professional advice or services to the individual reader. The ideas, procedures, and suggestions contained in this book are not intended to substitute for consulting with your physician. All matters regarding your health require medical supervision. Neither the author nor the publisher shall be liable or responsible for any claim of loss or damage arising from any information or suggestion in this book.

The recipes contained in this book are to be followed exactly as written. The publisher is not responsible for your specific health or allergy needs that may require medical supervision. The publisher is not responsible for any adverse reactions to the recipes contained in this book.

While the author has made every effort to provide accurate telephone numbers, Internet addresses, and other contact information at the time of publication, neither the publisher nor the author assumes any responsibility for errors or changes that occur after publication. Further, the publisher does not have any control over and does not assume any responsibility for third-party websites or their content.

Links

Throughout this book I have provided internet links to resources which are identified as <u>underlined</u> words, with the exception of subheadings. To keep these web addresses simple for the purpose of the printed version of this book, or electronic book readers that do not have web-browsers, I have created a master page for these links at https://www.healthybraintoolbox.com/links.

About the Author

Ken Sharlin, MD, MPH, IFMCP, is a board-certified neurologist, consultant, functional medicine practitioner, author, and speaker. He received his medical degrees from Emory University, and his functional medicine certification through The Institute for Functional Medicine. He is the #1 best-selling author of *The Healthy Brain Toolbox: Neurologist-Proven Strategies to Improve Memory Loss and Protect Your Aging Brain*, and of numerous essays that have appeared in media internationally. Dr. Sharlin is a 3-time Ironman Triathlon finisher who made his story of personal transformation the launching point of his career when he shifted gears from a conventional neurology practice to a holistic, lifestyle-medicine-oriented approach. Using the action plan presented in his book, Dr. Sharlin and his team have witnessed the reversal of illnesses that are supposed to be chronic and progressive, and in some cases fatal. He practices general neurology, conducts clinical research, and directs his functional medicine program, *Brain Tune Up!*, through his clinic, Sharlin Health and Neurology, located in Ozark, MO.

Follow Dr. Sharlin on Facebook and Twitter. Subscribe to his YouTube channel. Learn more about his *Brain Tune Up!* program and subscribe to his newsletter at his website.

Acknowledgements

Because of my wife's encouragement and support, I took the big leap to change my trajectory as a practicing neurologist. Thank you, Valerie, with all my heart, for helping me find my purpose. I would also like to express my appreciation to my entire office staff, and my *Brain Tune Up!* team, including Cāllie, Chuck, Angela, Amy, Merry, and Andrew. Gratitude also to my mentors, Dr. Terry Wahls, Dr. Norm Shealy, and the late Dr. John Stone. I want to recognize the pioneers of functional medicine, including Dr. Jeffrey Bland and Dr. David Perlmutter, without whom this would not be possible. Finally, thank you to all of my patients, who have allowed me the privilege of sharing in their own hero's journeys.

Praise for Dr. Ken Sharlin

"*I love his writing — the actionable, but outside-of-the-typical supplement-box, items we can engage ourselves and advise our patients to do. It's high time for more nuanced thinking in this arena. I'm thrilled that we've got such a cool functional neurologist in our midst.*"

—Kara Fitzgerald, ND, IFMCP,
Physician & Clinic Director (The Sandy Hook Clinic),
author of *Methylation Diet & Lifestyle* and *Case Studies in Integrative and Functional Medicine*, Faculty member at The Institute for Functional Medicine

"*Dr. Sharlin is a board-certified neurologist with expertise in helping people restore the health and vitality of their brains for many years. He is an outstanding clinician, an effective educator, speaker, and a gifted writer. He has my most enthusiastic support for his message to the world. There is hope for those with neurological issues!*"

—Terry L. Wahls, MD, Physician,
Researcher, Speaker, and author of *The Wahls Protocol: How I Beat MS Using Paleo Principles and Functional Medicine* and *The Wahls Protocol Cooking for Life*

"I've had the pleasure of working with Dr. Sharlin as a radio show host and a wellness magazine publisher. It quickly became clear to me that he is an excellent communicator, caring physician and healer of the highest caliber. It therefore came as no surprise that Dr. Sharlin would write a book that captures his extensive knowledge and experience walking with his patients on the path to sustained wellness using functional medicine. The subject is important and timely. In this volume, Dr. Sharlin explains the architecture of the brain, how to heal from disease, and practical strategies to reverse cognitive decline and prevent illness, all in an approachable and engaging manner. Since our neurological health in large part determines our quality of life, I can't think of a more important read for people of all ages."

—Sandra Guy Malhotra, PhD,
Owner and Editor-in-Chief of *Regenerate* magazine,
former host of the *Generation Regeneration* radio show on
VoiceAmerica Radio

"Although Dr. Sharlin is a board-certified neurologist (he was an undergraduate English major at Kenyon College), he utilizes his keen storytelling skills to unravel complex illnesses. For the reader, Dr. Sharlin creates a strong literary bedside manner to unravel medical mysteries in a style that is both helpful and hopeful. By redefining the science of healing through the power of common sense, The Healthy Brain Toolbox is a prescription for a healthier lifestyle."

—George M. Freeman, veteran journalist,
writer, and editor of *Ozarks Living* magazine

Table of Contents

PART 2
THE STRATEGIES

Foreword

by Terry Wahls, MD, IFMCP

Whether you are a practicing clinician, a patient with a brain problem, or the family member of someone with a brain-related problem, this book will give you a new set of tools to better understand and address brain-related health challenges.

When I was in medical school on the neurology rotation, we took careful histories, did thorough physical examinations, and tried to pinpoint the precise location in the brain where the problem was. It was a fun intellectual challenge, trying to predict what the brain imaging would show. But once we knew the origin, there was little to offer patients, which is why we students nicknamed neurology "diagnose, and then adios."

I wanted to be able to offer treatment that could make a difference, so I went into internal medicine, where we could prescribe medication to help our patients. We knew that most diseases were tied to improper biochemical processes in our cells, caused by the DNA. We trusted scientists to unravel the physiology and improper biochemistry and design new drugs to correct malfunctions. Our job as clinicians was to learn about the newest drugs that could be used to correct the biochemical processes and prescribe them accordingly.

Each year, we have ever more potent drugs, but the societal burden of poor health grows. More and more people are diagnosed with diabetes, which increases the risk for both stroke and cognitive decline. There are more people diagnosed with chronic headaches, fibromyalgia, and Parkinson's each year, and more children and young people diagnosed with multiple sclerosis and other autoimmune conditions at younger and younger ages.

Why is this happening to us? Are the increasing rates of these health problems due to our DNA? I was trained in medical school to blame someone's poor health on their DNA. I was taught to diagnose the problem quickly and start my patients on the newest, latest drugs--that is the way I practiced medicine for years, and it is the way most physicians practice still. But are our genes the root of these neurological problems, or is there something else going on?

Genes do matter. Scientists have identified over 200 genes that increase the risk, ever so slightly, for developing multiple sclerosis. The vast majority of risk for developing multiple sclerosis, however, is the result of a complex interaction between one's DNA and a lifetime of diet quality, physical activity level, stress level, and smoking status. The same is true for most chronic health problems, including neurological ones. It is not our DNA that creates our health problems, but rather it is the interaction of our DNA and our diet and lifestyle choices, including environmental exposures.

This is the best possible news for clinicians, patients, and their families. This means that we have more areas of opportunities to help our patients reduce the risk of developing a neurological (or medical) problem, and many more ways beyond drug-based treatments to decrease the severity of the symptoms and improve the response to treatment.

In *The Healthy Brain Toolbox*, you will learn more about how to approach brain-related symptoms and how the major organ systems contribute to improving or worsening brain health. This book will bring you new insights into the biochemistry of life, what supports proper biochemistry, and what kinds of things in a person's diet, lifestyle, and environment can derail it.

The good news is that for many, this type of approach can yield remarkable results, even when the conventional treatments have failed. I am one of those people. I have progressive MS, and had seen the best doctors at one of the best MS centers in the country, but still experienced 7 years of steady decline, despite taking the newest drugs. When I began using the same kinds of principles that Dr. Sharlin will teach you in *The Healthy Brain Toolbox* to address the root causes of why my brain's biochemistry was malfunctioning, the totally unexpected happened: I stopped getting worse. Even more surprising, I got better. The fatigue was replaced with more and more energy. The brain fog was replaced with mental clarity. My tilt-recline wheelchair was replaced with canes. Then the canes were put away and I was biking again.

This book is filled with hope and possibilities. Clinicians will learn a new way to think about their patients with chronic health problems. Patients and families will gain tools to begin taking charge of their health. This *Toolbox* will help you take charge of your diet and lifestyle choices, create a better environment for your brain cells, and make your brain healthier, happier, and more functional. Are you ready to get your life back? Dr. Sharlin will show you the way!

Terry Wahls, MD, IFMCP
Clinical Professor of Medicine and Neurology, University of Iowa
Author, *The Wahls Protocol: How I Beat Progressive MS
Using Functional Medicine and Paleo Principles* and
The Wahls Protocol Cooking for Life

PART 1
THE SCIENCE

CHAPTER 1

Houston, We Have a Problem!

How to Think Outside the Box to
Solve a Global Health Crisis

"We must let go of the life we have planned so as to accept the one that is waiting for us."
—Joseph Campbell, mythologist and writer

The statistics are staggering. According to Alzheimer's Disease International, someone in the world develops dementia every three seconds. Worldwide, nearly 50 million people have Alzheimer's or a related dementia. In the United States alone, more than five million Americans are living with Alzheimer's, where it is the sixth leading cause of death. The growth rate is steep. Although hope may be on the horizon, there is currently no FDA-approved treatment to prevent these changes or reverse the course of this devastating condition. In the U.S., Alzheimer's prevalence is expected to reach 16 million by the year 2050.

The Centers for Disease Control and Prevention released a study in 2011 looking at households in 13 states, and found that in 12.6%, at least one adult had memory loss or confusion. Even more concerning, in 5.4% (1 in 20 households), *all the adults* had experienced increased memory loss or confusion[1]. Sporadic Alzheimer's makes up the large majority, currently 5.5 out of the 5.7 million Americans. The term "sporadic" suggests that the development of Alzheimer's disease cannot be predicted by genetics alone. The evidence points toward environmental factors as having a major role in determining the risk of Alzheimer's disease. Armed with the information gained from this book, it may be possible — for those willing to embark on the journey — to utilize environment-altering strategies to avoid memory loss and protect the aging brain.

The numbers concerning other diseases affecting the adult brain are equally astonishing. Worldwide, neurological disorders are now the leading cause of disability. The latest information suggests there are 1 million people in the United States with multiple sclerosis and 2.3 million people globally[2]. *The Journal of the American Medical Association* published "A Call to Action," because Parkinson's disease is the fastest growing of the neurological disorders, with a growth rate surpassing that of Alzheimer's. According to the authors, the number of people worldwide with Parkinson's is expected to double from 6.9 million in 2015 to 14.2 million in 2040.

Consider a neurological condition that affects the brain at all ages. Over 15% of all adults complain about severe headaches or migraines, and the prevalence among women is more than twice as high as among men. It is the third most common and the sixth most disabling illness in the world, with healthcare and lost productivity costs associated with migraines estimated to be as high as $36 billion annually, in the United States[3].

Chronic pain, largely under the control of the brain, is another devastating condition It is the most common cause of long-term disability. Conditions like fibromyalgia affect an estimated 10 million people in the United States, and anyone who has this illness will attest that it involves far more than tenderness of muscles. Brain fog, depression, numbness, gut and bladder dysfunction, fatigue, loss of appetite, and many other symptoms characterize this devastating, total body illness.

Here are some of the patients I have seen in my Brain Tune Up! clinic:

About 6 years ago, when Janice was 56, her family noticed she was having problems with her memory. At the time, she was working as a bookkeeper in the family business. The early signs were subtle. She would repeat stories, questions, or forget conversations she had. She might say she was going to get groceries, then forget to do so. She made mistakes bookkeeping. Her family physician attributed the problem to "senior moments." When the mistakes became more frequent, she was sent for an MRI of her brain to rule out stroke. No stroke was identified, but further investigation included a spinal fluid examination, and this test revealed abnormal levels of proteins consistent with Alzheimer's disease.

Richard, at 76 years old, came to see me for mild cognitive impairment. He is a retired investment banker who had experienced the abrupt onset of depression, anxiety, and "brain fog" after his surgery for benign prostatic hypertrophy, three months earlier. He took medicine for blood pressure, cholesterol, and to help him control the bladder incontinence which followed his surgery. His Montreal Cognitive Assessment score (a measure of several dimensions of memory and thinking) was 23 out of 30 (normal is greater than or equal to 26). Richard needs further evaluation.

William, a preacher in his mid 70's, started to have trouble speaking, at the pulpit. His symptoms progressed over two years and got so bad he had to retire from his work. He would get stuck on words or stop in the middle of sentences. In addition, he has a sleep disorder called Obstructive Sleep Apnea. His wife says the abnormal breathing went on for years before he agreed to get checked by a doctor. She observed loud snoring and pauses in his breath. He now uses an assistive device at night called CPAP (Continuous Positive Airway Pressure). William had a genetic analysis that revealed two copies of a gene known to place him at high risk for Alzheimer's disease, called ApoE4.

Tim was a 48 year old carpenter who, over the past 5 years, had noticed a decline in his memory. The problem had gotten much worse in the months leading up to his neurology appointment and had been interfering with his work. He had trouble with attention, focus, and concentration. He felt like his mind was "short circuiting." He struggled with adding numbers, normally not a problem. Like William, he had trouble with word-finding. It had become a source of embarrassment. Sometimes the wrong word would come out, and his co-workers would laugh at him when he made these mistakes. He had also gotten lost while driving. Over the years, he had experienced several emotional blows, including the unexpected death of his father when he was 12, and then that of his stepfather a few years later. He had a difficult marriage that threw him into a state of depression, in the years leading up to divorce and for several years afterwards. He had been a welder, a crop duster, and most recently a carpenter, and with each of these jobs, there was the potential for exposure to toxins like metals, pesticides, paints, varnishes, and mold.

Regardless of your reason for picking up this book, it is never too early to think about protecting your brain. The vignettes I share are not limited to memory, nor are they restricted to older age. Tim, whose narrative I just discussed, is 48 years old. Eric and Karen, who follow, are 59 and 32 years old, and their stories are about ALS and fibromyalgia, respectively. Other conditions, like migraine and multiple sclerosis, can affect a person at any age, and both have the potential to cause a tremendous amount of disability. So, fasten your seatbelt. You are about to embark on a journey to discover a new way of thinking about the brain. Travel light. The road will not be easy. But along the way you will add some powerful tools to your toolbox to carry with you through the rest of your life!

Now, let's meet Eric.

Eric had a successful career in the corporate world. He was offered an entry-level job with a multinational company when he graduated from college. Over time, he reached Group President, and might have become CEO, but had to retire unexpectedly. He was in his mid-fifties and still active. He thought he was healthy. But he noticed, when running with his son, that his left leg felt weak, and he had a tendency to turn his foot. He visited an orthopedist, who thought he might have a problem with his lumbar spine. A second opinion from a neurologist identified the presence of overactive reflexes in his legs (the response when the knees and ankles are tapped with a rubber reflex hammer) and a nerve test, called electromyography, showed the problem to be more widespread. There was deterioration of the nerves that controlled the muscles of his arms and legs, and those along his spine. The doctor was concerned he might have Amyotrophic Lateral Sclerosis, and a trip to a prestigious medical center confirmed the diagnosis. Eric came to see me because his quarterly follow up visits with his regular neurologist focused on determining if he was in decline, rather than offering hope and common sense science-based options.

Karen is a registered nurse who worked until the birth of her now 15-month-old child. Her symptoms started post-partum. She developed neck and upper back pain followed by tingling in the right shoulder blade area that would come on, last a few minutes, then go away, triggered by activity, such as walking. The symptoms started in March 2016, then in May, two months later, she underwent Lasik surgery for her vision, which she described as "always blurry." Though the procedure was declared successful by her ophthalmologist, she began "battling" with her eyes from that time forward. They felt dry, and she continued to have problems with her vision. In October 2016, a sense of muscle exhaustion in her right arm developed, which eventually spread to the face and leg on the same side, then to both sides of the body. She had numbness as if it were below the skin, then she started hurting everywhere. She went to her doctor. Initially, the thought was that

Karen had multiple sclerosis or another autoimmune disease. Her brain MRI was normal, which made MS unlikely, but her blood tests were positive for two antibodies associated with autoimmunity. When she visited with a rheumatologist, he felt like the blood tests were spurious, and there was no disease he could attribute to the results. That doctor suggested consultation with a neurologist. She followed through and the neurologist explored depression and fibromyalgia as possible diagnoses. He suggested treatment with a drug approved for both conditions, but Karen declined the offer, and came to see me instead.

How are we to frame this information in our own lives? More than likely, you or someone you know suffers from a condition affecting the brain. We go to the doctor, our point of authority, and tests are run. We hope for an answer, a diagnosis, but too often the treatment fails to meet our expectations for options to return to a state of resilient health. This book will explore some of the current and emerging evidence that there are tools each of us can use to prevent memory loss and protect the aging brain. Though specific guidance will be provided, the book is an invitation to join me on a journey to explore a new way of thinking about health, medicine, and how the brain works. *Warning: the first part is pretty sciency.* But I encourage you to stick with it.

The information I will share is based on functional medicine, a specific approach to healthcare that is gaining ground in the United States and worldwide. Functional medicine, in turn, was born out of the science of systems biology. If you're confused, don't worry. All of this will be explained in the pages to come. So, while prescriptive recommendations are offered for the taking, you, the reader, are discouraged from skipping to the end to consume this information right away. Instead, by following the sequence in which the book is written, you will discover treasures in these pages that compel you to examine your innermost self, and to an opportunity to experience a transformation that might change your life — as it did mine — forever.

To unravel these strategies to avoid memory loss and protect your aging brain, it is first necessary to change the way you think about how illness occurs, and how we in western medicine have organized our thinking around disease management. For example, I am a neurologist, which means that I treat diseases that affect the nervous system. The nervous system is defined as the brain, brainstem, spinal cord, nerve roots, peripheral nerves, the interface between nerve and muscle called the neuromuscular junction, and the muscles themselves. Similarly, there are doctors whose specialties focus on the heart (cardiologists), the digestive system (gastroenterologists), the bones (orthopedists), the hormone systems (endocrinologists), and so forth. These divisions suggest that the body works by organ systems that do not connect to one another and that the diseases, as expressed, occur exclusively within those organ systems, while leaving the rest of the body unaffected or uninvolved. This is not true of the heart, gut, bones, or hormones, and it is certainly not true of the brain.

The new paradigm is to think about a holistic system, with each part connected to and influenced by another part, and how each of them is affected by environmental factors that are largely under our control. To further explore this shift, I would like to share with you my personal journey.

CHAPTER 2

I am a Product of My Generation

The Truth About How I Got Here

"An autobiography is not about pictures; it's about the stories; it's about honesty and as much truth as you can tell."
—Boris Becker, professional tennis player

I grew up in New Jersey in an upper middle-class family. My mother was a special education teacher and my father a pediatrician. I was exposed to the arts at an early age, and enjoyed numerous books. I even browsed through *The New York Times Sunday Edition* over a "good" cup of coffee from a remarkably young age. I have a younger brother and sister, and my parents cared deeply about the quality of our upbringing. They traveled with us and introduced us to numerous sports and experiences. They encouraged us to be active in whatever we happened to be passionate about. By every account, my life has been privileged, and I am grateful.

I am a product of my time, my community, and my family. Television was an important form of entertainment in our home. Aside from the classic TV shows of the 60s and 70s, regularly aired commercials suggested the best ways to live my life. Unconsciously, I submitted to all sorts of messaging, including recommendations on how I should eat. I learned about breakfast cereals promoted by a cartoon ship captain, pulpy "fresh" orange juice in a carton, milk to make my bones strong, nutritious whole grain bread, sandwich meats with a first name, soups that were "Mmm . . . Good!" and America's favorite sugar-sweetened soft drink that assured me, "It's the real thing, baby." Of course, food advertising was not limited to television. Everywhere I looked, examples were being set for what constituted the standard American diet. It became second nature, part of my being. I remember when the restaurant known for the big, golden arches first opened in my town. "Organic" was not on the table, nor in our vocabulary. When it came to margarine, butter was not better. My family, friends, and community enjoyed similar food, and we thought that it was good.

Fortunately, I still spent plenty of time outside, as a child. I grew up in a place and an era when parents worried a little less about their children during the after-school hours. I rode my bike everywhere. I had after-school activities or I spent time with my best friend, Victor. Summers were enjoyed at the local community pool, day and sleep away camp. There was summer swim league. When I got older, I worked as a lifeguard. If the weather allowed, I spent time outside throwing a baseball or kicking a soccer ball. On a cold or rainy day, I might be inside listening to music, playing guitar, or designing spaceships for our imaginary fleet of Federation Starships modeled from the original Star Trek. By all standards, I was going through life the only way I knew. It felt safe and it felt natural.

The 1980s were my college and medical school years, and a lot has changed since that time. When I think about the community in which I lived in central New Jersey, and the people who were 10-20 years older than I am now, who had normal lives back then, about 15% now have Alzheimer's disease. We now think that changes in the brain which lead to Alzheimer's begin more than a decade before the onset of illness[4]. Who would have suspected? Could it have been predicted? If changes had been made then, might things now be different?

There are several risk factors for progressive memory loss, which include obesity, high blood pressure, diabetes, sleep apnea, stress, sedentary lifestyle, and social isolation, among others. All of these are risk factors for Alzheimer's disease.

A risk factor is a biologically plausible characteristic or exposure that increases the possibility of contracting an illness or disease. If we track the prevalence of these risk factors into the first two decades of the 21st century, we find there has been a remarkable rise over time. In 2008, obesity affected 9.8% of men and 13.8% of women in the world, compared with 4.8% for men and 7.9% for women in 1980[5]. The problem is far more common in the United States, where more than one-third of U.S. adults suffer from obesity.

Obesity is tied to the risk of high blood pressure, diabetes, and Obstructive Sleep Apnea. When it comes to high blood pressure, data from the National Health and Nutrition Examination Survey indicate that the overall age-adjusted prevalence of hypertension among U.S. adults is 29.0% (2011-2012)[6]. Both the percentage and the number of people with diabetes have dramatically risen in the United States. Centers for Disease Control estimate that approximately 9.40% of Americans have been diagnosed with diabetes (2015), representing 30.3 million Americans[7]. The National Healthy Sleep Awareness Project published data, in a 2013 edition of the *American Journal of Epidemiology*, on the increased prevalence of sleep apnea, a condition characterized by long pauses in breathing while a person is asleep. It was then estimated that at least 25 million adults in the United States suffer from this condition[8]. Obstructive sleep apnea contributes to the risk of heart attack and heart failure, in addition to disorders of memory loss such as Alzheimer's Disease, and premature death.

Stress, physical activity, and social connection are also closely associated with brain health and disease. In January 2012, the American

Psychological Association released a report entitled Stress in America: Our Health at Risk[9]. Acknowledging the strong link between stress and overall health, the report suggested that the concern about stress and health is especially critical among adults age 50 and older. The 2011 estimate of the number or percentage of Americans who report extreme stress was 22%, as defined on a 10-point scale where extreme stress was rated an eight, nine, or ten. Physical inactivity (defined as the percentage of adults who report doing no physical activity or exercise other than their regular job in the past 30 days) characterizes 22.6% of Americans overall, with the least healthy state being Mississippi, where the prevalence of physical inactivity reaches 31.6%, based on current data[10]. Physical inactivity affects more women, more Hispanic and black adults, older adults, adults living in the South, adults with lower educational attainment, and those with lower income. Finally, the prevalence of social isolation remains a major health problem for older adults. Social isolation (defined as a state in which the individual lacks a sense of belonging socially or engagement with others) may be as high as 43% in older adults[11]. Loneliness and social isolation are both linked to Alzheimer's disease.

Who are we, and how did we get here? I shared a small part of my childhood in New Jersey, and it turns out that local context does shape us in ways beyond what one might expect from the programs encoded by our genes. Science now tells us that our environment influences the expression of our genes, turning on those promoting health, and silencing those that promote disease. In the end, our world is defined by our own traditions, beliefs, and habits. When I was growing up, we had an expression: "It is what it is." This is the trajectory that allows us to go through life blindly guided by our unconscious selves. What the reader will soon discover is that to avoid memory loss and protect the aging brain, we need to step out of this reality and challenge some of the notions about our own lives that we think are unalterable, or beyond our individual control.

CHAPTER 3

The Apple Can Land Far from the Tree, If You Give it a Push

How A Conventionally-Trained Doctor Turned into a Functional Medicine Fanatic

"Every new adjustment is a crisis in self-esteem."
—Eric Hoffer, philosopher and writer

I attended medical school at Emory University School of Medicine. It was a struggle to get there. Medical school entrance was, as it is now, highly competitive, and I was not a straight A student with perfect medical school entrance examination board scores. Early in my college years, I had serendipitously come across a magazine article featuring a physician-writer whose name was John Stone. Dr. Stone was a dean and cardiologist at Emory University, and a well-published poet and essayist. I had a passion for creative writing from a young age, and although I knew I wanted to become a doctor, I struggled with what I thought were polar interests — my interest in writing and my desire to practice medicine.

I identified so strongly with Dr. Stone that I collected some poems I had written, put them in an envelope with a personal note about myself, my interest in writing, and my desire to be a doctor, and sent them to him. I was delighted when several weeks later, I received a package in the mail with a response from Dr. Stone, indicating he had read my poems and encouraging me to keep writing and stay in touch. I was a student at Kenyon College in central Ohio, a school famous for its Department of English, its prestigious literary journal, and the long lineage of writers who had passed through its hallways as faculty and students, and naturally, I was an English major.

I thrived in the humanities at Kenyon, where the goal of the liberal arts education can be summed up in the phrase "to seek the truth." There, I also became familiar with the writing of neurologist Dr. Oliver Sacks, whose book, *The Man Who Mistook His Wife for a Hat*, challenged my own notions about reality and inspired me to become a neurologist. I read the poetry of Dr. William Carlos Williams, the great American poet from Paterson, New Jersey. I enjoyed the plays of Anton Chekhov, the essays of Lewis Thomas and Richard Selzer, the short stories of Ferrol Sams, and the novels of Walker Percy, all also doctors. When it came time to write my thesis for the department of English, I was encouraged to explore the physician-as-writer, with a focus on Dr. Stone's work. I traveled to Atlanta with a cassette recorder and several blank tapes to interview Dr. Stone in preparation for my thesis.

Following graduation, after a year living in Washington, D.C., I moved to Atlanta to begin a master's degree in public health while I worked on my medical school entrance application. I was fortunate to be offered a place at Emory, and I eagerly started my journey toward becoming a doctor the summer of 1988. I was ready to embrace everything that I would be taught, without question. My first year of medical school was spent studying normal anatomy and how the body works. This meant courses in anatomy, physiology, microbiology, biochemistry, behavioral science, histology (the study of tissue under the microscope), and neuroscience.

Beginning the second year, I was given a stethoscope, other examination instruments, my first doctor's bag, and a white coat. This marked the beginning of my journey into care of the sick patient. I would learn how to take a history and perform a physical examination. My classes now focused on pharmacology and pathology, and centered around diseases of the different organ system from the heart to the lungs, kidneys, digestive tract, muscles, nervous system, and hormone-producing glands. The transition between the first and the second years was like flipping a light switch from on to off, from health to disease.

We went from a study of perfect health and normal function to a study of illness and disease, without taking time to understand the transition between these two states. In my third and fourth years, during the clinical rotations on different medical specialty services, as well as pediatrics and general adult medicine, I would learn that the options for treatment were medications or surgery with support from physical, occupational, and speech therapists. No other avenues were considered. Illness was viewed more as a fact of life than a process in which a previously healthy individual experienced a variety of triggering events through their lifetimes, that ultimately led them on a trajectory to illness. There was no consideration of the possibility that this trajectory could be changed.

Following graduation from medical school, I spent the next several years training in general medicine and neurology. This further reinforced my thinking. Beyond antibiotics and diseases known to be self-limited, like the common cold, the only time I embraced the idea that a medical condition could be resolved was when I echoed the words of my surgery friends, who would say, "To cut is to cure." I finished my neurology training in 1998 with this notion firmly embedded in my psyche. This was my reality, and it would be many years before this reality was challenged.

In the year 2000, I moved my family to Springfield, Missouri, where I took a job as staff neurologist and director of the stroke program at Mercy Hospital. For the next several years, my work in both the hospital and clinic settings focused on treating the acutely sick and the chronically ill. Stroke, for example, was discussed in terms of primary or secondary prevention, in addition to the care of the patient with an acute stroke in the hospital. Primary prevention meant that it might be possible to prevent a person from ever having a stroke in the first place. Unfortunately, there was little my specialty of neurology had to offer in this arena. The strategy for secondary prevention, focused on preventing a second stroke after a first occurred, was to prescribe aspirin or a blood thinner, screen the carotid arteries for major blockages, look at the heart for abnormalities that would raise the risk of stroke, lower cholesterol and blood pressure with medications, refer to the primary care doctor for better control of diabetes, and encourage our patients to quit cigarette smoking, sometimes with the aid of another medication. Yet, how common is it to have a second stroke? According to the American Heart Association, of the 795,000 strokes that occur every year, about 185,000 (1 in 4) are in individuals who have had a previous stroke[12]. Poor statistics. Should we be more aggressive with medication?

In a study of the effects of intensive glucose lowering in type II diabetics published in the *New England Journal of Medicine* on June 12, 2008, researchers found that aggressive blood sugar lowering among diabetics resulted in increased deaths among patients, compared to the control group, and the study was halted. Similarly, the *British Medical Journal* published in 2016 featured an article in which aggressive blood pressure lowering (less than 140 millimeters of mercury in patients with diabetes) resulted in increased risk of cardiovascular death, with no observed benefit.

Related to these observations is a statistic known as "the number needed to treat." It is a measure of the effectiveness of any treatment within the population, and reflects the number of people that need to be treated with a particular medication to prevent an endpoint such as heart attack, stroke, or death. As a doctor who prescribed medication to my patients, what I did not realize and therefore did not tell them, is that more likely than not, the drug recommended would fail to prevent the event for which it was being prescribed in the first place.

For example, if we ask how many people need to be treated with blood pressure medication to prevent one premature death? The answer is 125 people. If we ask how many need to be treated to prevent one stroke? The answer is 67. To prevent one heart attack, treat 100[13]. So with medication alone, it is more likely that my patients will not benefit than that they will. In fact, it is probably more likely that they will experience a side effect from the medication than any benefit at all. Even more disturbing, in light of recent adjustments to the guidelines that define thresholds for treatment of conditions like high cholesterol and high blood pressure was a report released in 2012 by the Cochrane Collaboration, suggesting that treatment for mild hypertension showed no difference between treated and untreated individuals in heart attack, stroke, and death[14].

Over the next several years, I built a practice focusing on conditions that included migraines, fibromyalgia, multiple sclerosis, epilepsy, Parkinson's disease, amyotrophic lateral sclerosis, Alzheimer's disease and other disorders of memory loss. The economic demands of medicine required that I, like other doctors, saw an increasing number of patients per day in my clinic, while applying protocols which, while rational, were often mechanistic and had more to do with matching a pill for an ill than understanding the unique stories of each of my patients and the factors that contributed to their trajectories of illness. I became increasingly frustrated with the profession I had chosen.

In my personal life, things were different. In 2006, my wife Valerie, whose marketing job for a local hospital includes organizing adventurous activities for older adults, announced that she was starting a bicycle club. Even though this was for work, she thought that bicycling was something we could do together. I had been a bike enthusiast, but somewhere between medical school, postgraduate training, and my early days of employment, I lost my connection with my bicycle and no longer owned one. This meant, of course, that we would need to buy bicycles, and after I got over my initial sticker shock at the fancy carbon-framed bicycles with their super lightweight components, I settled on what I thought was something more reasonable for both of us.

Soon, a rekindled interest would grow into marked enthusiasm as we conquered rides of increasingly longer distances. We started bicycle teams and trained together. Rides of 28-mile distances led to 45 and 64-mile rides, then eventually 100 miles, the MS 150 and the Iowa Register's Great Bicycle Ride Across Iowa (RAGBRAI). As my training progressed, my body changed. And after a few years of long-distance riding, I yearned for a greater challenge.

It was common for pharmaceutical representatives to visit my office. Two of them who came in regularly shared with me their experiences with the sport of triathlon. This single race consists of three separate legs: a swim, followed by a bicycle race, followed by a run. This seemed nearly impossible for me at the time, but I was fascinated with the idea that it might be something I could accomplish. One day, while visiting a local bicycle shop, I saw a flyer advertising a youth triathlon. In the fine print, it said that parents could participate in a demonstration heat if they had one child registered.

My son Gabe was 16 years old, and a good athlete, and I asked him if he might be interested in entering the race together. He agreed, and with little knowledge of how to train (except that it would be necessary to spend time in the swimming pool and building my run endurance, neither of which I was accustomed to), both of us worked out enthusiastically. Race day arrived, and we were both transformed by the experience of our successful completion of the event. I went on to do two more triathlons that summer, and that was just the beginning.

I participated in races of increasingly greater length and eventually completed three Ironman triathlons in Canada and Mexico, two marathons, and many other racing events in between. In order to successfully complete the triathlon, especially the 140.6 miles distance that is the Ironman triathlon, I learned that a training plan consisted of more than well-written or well-executed workouts. Mindset is critical, and attention to quality sleep, nutrition, stress resilience, and community were of equal importance. My patients were aware of my passion for cycling, running, and swimming, and I knew that these efforts were transforming my life both physically and spiritually.

While I built resilience, my patients with chronic diseases — my Alzheimer's, Parkinson's, and multiple sclerosis patients — often deteriorated. To remain relatively stable, my MS patients had to take powerful disease-modifying drugs, endure their side effects and complications, two of which place them at risk for a devastating brain infection called Progressive Multifocal Leukoencephalopathy. Other drugs can cause liver failure or trigger thoughts of suicide.

The problems were not limited to MS. My migraine patients and my patients with fibromyalgia had no choice but to settle for medications proven to help control symptoms while not addressing the underlying causes of their illnesses. The conventional treatment toolbox, at best, provided short-term benefit only. Many patients continued to deteriorate over time, and this was the expectation, a silent agreement between us that disease was inevitable, and most treatments were a temporizing solution to a long-term problem or a long-term commitment with no resolution in sight. I would be there to pick up the pieces or to offer my condolences to families, when my patients died.

One day, while listening to a triathlon-related podcast, the host was interviewing a physician (another neurologist) who said that he was on faculty at The Institute for Functional Medicine, where physicians studied and learned to treat patients by addressing the root causes of disease. My ears perked up and I investigated this newfound path, in hope that it might provide insight into the struggle I had been experiencing in my profession. The more I learned about functional medicine, the more I came to believe that functional medicine held the answers I was seeking in my career. But was I up for the challenge? I was already in my late 40s. The idea of going to school to learn a new kind of medicine, to change the way I thought about illness and my role as a doctor, was exciting but came with a skepticism and hesitation, as well.

CHAPTER 4

Inflammation and Oxidative Stress

Unearthing the Root Causes of Chronic Disease

"I think that any time of great pain is a time of transformation, a fertile time to plant new seeds."

—Debbie Ford, writer and motivational speaker

As you dive into this chapter, I am going to take one more shot across the bow, as I did in Chapter 1. The reader will find this chapter, and the next two, to be fairly technical. But they contain information about the underlying processes at work in the body and build a foundation for the solutions offered in **Part 2**. To get the most out of this book, and avoid the trap of a formulaic prescription, it is necessary to be grounded in the principles which underlie the approach I am going to share with you. These principles give life to the ideas and provide you the tools to go beyond the boundaries of this book, into the expanding universe of knowledge that is functional medicine.

One of the things Dr. Stone taught me early on was that the word doctor is derived from the Latin word *docere*, which means "to teach." Doctor as teacher is a great image and ideal to follow, and it carried me through medical school and post-graduate training. In the hospital setting, patients are cared for by teams of doctors with an established pecking order — the medical student is at the bottom, followed by the first year post-graduate, called an intern, then residents of ascending years. Depending on the length or type program, this is followed by physicians who have completed residency but are continuing to get additional specialized education and experience, called fellows, and then finally the attending physician.

I am grateful for the many teachers I had during those years, including the patients themselves, who allowed me to learn from them when I was the lowest man on the totem pole. By the time they saw me the patients had told their histories and submitted to physical exams several times already. In my clinic practice, probably the part I enjoy the most about patient evaluations is the opportunity I have to share information with my patient after a comprehensive history and physical, and gathering of test results, so that the patient can better understand the problem that they are having, and we can work together toward an acceptable solution. Every patient is different, even when their conditions are the same.

The degree I got from Emory is Medical Doctor or MD, and this has been termed "allopathic medicine" to distinguish it from the degree of DO, received by physicians who graduate from schools of osteopathy. The term allopathic medicine, interestingly, was coined by the father of homeopathic medicine, Dr. Samuel Hahnemann, in 1810, to describe an approach to medicine that uses remedies, which produce effects in healthy patients that are different from the effects produced by the disease itself. This is in contrast with the homeopaths, who use substances that cause similar effects to the symptoms of a disease they might be treating. But in the end, the term was invented as a way to hurl criticism by suggesting the main approach of allopathic medicine is to target symptoms, rather than the underlying causes of the disease.

This is not entirely true, of course. But in many cases — at least, when it comes to the care of patients on a day to day basis — many of the treatments do focus on the downstream effects, such as ways to lower high blood pressure, high cholesterol, or high blood sugar, without addressing why the disease occurred in the first place. Still other treatments are focused on altering the behavior of the immune system, and while they are more upstream, they still do not address the problem at the root cause level, meaning, what caused the immune system to misbehave in the first place.

Early on, I learned that functional medicine would teach me how to investigate those important individual "whys" while at the same time emphasizing the whole person. It focuses on the patient as much as the disease. In functional medicine, the process of healing is one of empowerment through information and guidance. The most conventional medicine asks of patients is that they show up to appointments, fill their prescriptions, and take the drugs that have been prescribed. The drugs do the work. Functional medicine, on the other hand, is an active process that leads to transformation. To me, this is a much more exciting and rewarding way to practice medicine. But I had to get past the dogma of conventional medicine, and the fear of making this change, after so many years. Fortunately, I would have new mentors to accompany me.

Functional medicine uses the image of a tree to explain its approach to unraveling the way we think about disease and how we approach it from a treatment viewpoint. The organ systems or medical specialties can be thought of as the distant branches of the tree. As we move toward the main branches, and then the trunk, the image of the tree suggests that all diseases share common causes. Those two causes are: **inflammation** and **oxidative stress.**

INFLAMMATION

Inflammation is a complex process which involves the coordination of our immune systems — particularly our white blood cells — and importantly for our discussion, the chemical signals produced by tissues of the body called cytokines. Now, there are situations where acute inflammation can be dangerous, such as a severe allergic reaction, but if we think about it in more general terms, such as the area of inflammation that revolves around a small cut on the skin, this inflammation is playing a key role in controlling infection and, over time, healing the tissue. Here, inflammation is a normal and beneficial process. It is the body's response to injury. It helps to heal wounds. It is the body's defensive response to foreign invaders like viruses, bacteria, or parasites. In the brain, inflammation is even important for how our brains lay down memory (more on that, later). What matters for us is not whether or not inflammation is present, but its duration and intensity.

The environment that is not in balance, where inflammation is persistent, is an environment of chronic inflammation, and chronic inflammation has an entirely different effect on the body and brain. It will start to destroy healthy tissue. The pattern of chronic inflammation most pertinent to our discussion involves the resident immune cells in the brain, known as microglia, and those signaling molecules, cytokines.

In the brain, persistent inflammation of this nature does not have the cardinal signs of inflammation we might see around a bad cut on the skin, such as redness, pain, or swelling, but as it destroys healthy tissue over time, the result is a gradual pruning down of networks of brain cells, known as neurons, and then eventual destruction of the neurons themselves. If we think of memory as the complexity of nerve cell connections, called synapses, then the loss of synapses and destruction of neurons result in loss of memory, over time. It goes further, because neuroinflammation has been implicated in a wide variety of disorders affecting the brain, from Alzheimer's to Parkinson's disease, multiple sclerosis, amyotrophic lateral sclerosis, depression, chronic post-concussion syndromes (including Chronic Traumatic Encephalopathy), Post-Traumatic Stress Disorder, and others.

The most common cytokines involved in promotion of inflammation are Interleukin-1 beta, Interleukin-6, Tumor Necrosis Factor-alpha, and Interferon-gamma. The various impacts of these cytokines are diverse:

- They stimulate the immune cells to produce more pro-inflammatory cytokines;
- They activate microglia;
- They regulate growth factor activity;
- They influence synaptic strength and synaptic preservation;
- They influence growth of the key short-term memory area of the brain called the hippocampus;
- They stimulate progenitor stem cells to become new neurons; and
- They activate programmed cell death, a process called apoptosis.

Connecting microglia, cytokines, and neurons is a key protein known as Brain-Derived Neurotrophic Factor (BDNF). BDNF is a nerve growth factor involved in the development of neurons and their synapses. Additionally, it enhances neurotransmitter release. This is the chemical cross-talk that allows nerve cells to communicate with one another and the supportive cells (glia) in their environment. BDNF is a key player when it comes to preventing memory loss and protecting the aging brain, and it turns out that these cytokines affect the expression of BDNF.

OXIDATIVE STRESS

Like inflammation, oxidative stress is a normal byproduct of the chemistry of life. If we journey inside the cell, we find among its many parts the mitochondria. These critical organelles are responsible for producing the basic packet of energy that drives cellular reactions, called adenosine triphosphate, or ATP. The production of ATP begins when a cell breaks down glucose or fat, and through two processes known as the Krebs Cycle and Oxidative Phosphorylation, makes these substrates that hold substantial energy in their phosphate bonds. All this happens through the utilization of oxygen. Carbon dioxide and water are end-products in the manufacture of ATP, and to a lesser extent, reactive oxygen species.

When oxygen splits into single atoms with unpaired electrons, we call these products "free radicals." Free radicals will seek out other electrons so they can become a pair, which makes them highly reactive until that pairing is accomplished. Though not exclusive to mitochondria, they are, nevertheless, a major source of free radicals. If unchecked, these free radicals can harm important cellular structures like proteins, lipids, and even DNA itself. But under normal conditions, they can be managed through a variety of enzyme defense systems and exogenous antioxidants that come through food. Two of the more common oxygen-based free radicals are superoxide (two molecules of oxygen with an extra electron, O_2^-) and hydrogen peroxide (two molecules of hydrogen and two molecules of oxygen, H_2O_2). The two enzymes that reduce these free radicals into less damaging molecules are known as superoxide dismutase and catalase. Free radicals take the form of reactive oxygen and nitrogen species, and this is no mistake of nature. These free radicals play a key role in healthy cellular function when the cell is in a state of balance.

In mammals, the production of reactive oxygen species is antimicrobial against viruses, bacteria, and fungi. These oxidants are necessary for the maturation process of cellular structures, play a key role in intracellular signaling, destroy tumors, and induce cell division. The fact that excess oxidative stress plays a key role in numerous diseases throughout the body, including the brain, calls for a deeper understanding of the factors that drive oxidative stress. Like inflammation, oxidative stress can negatively impact the expression of BDNF. They go hand-in-hand, each feeding the other, in a manner that fuels the progression of disease.

When it comes to preventing memory loss and protecting the aging brain, the strategy is to identify the many ways we can balance inflammation and oxidative stress. To do so, it is necessary to travel further down the tree trunk, and ultimately into the depths of the soil, to the roots, and the seven biological systems that govern how the body actually functions as a whole. These systems are Assimilation, Defense & Repair, Energy, Biotransformation & Elimination, Transport, Communication, and Structural Integrity.

CHAPTER 5

The Seven Biological Systems

Imbalances in Functional Systems Affect One Another and Spark the Fire of Illness

"It is the harmony of the diverse parts, their symmetry, their happy balance; in a word it is all that introduces order, all that gives unity, that permits us to see clearly and to comprehend at once both the ensemble and the details."

—Henri Poincare, mathematician

The seven biological systems are different, as I have said, from the organ systems that are the main focus of conventional medicine. We treat the organ systems individually, with little regard to how they interact and affect one another. By contrast, a functional medicine approach recognizes that illness occurs as a result of imbalances within and between these systems. By identifying and mapping the specific imbalances, it opens the door to new strategies for management of disease at the root cause level. It allows us to see how perturbations in the system, triggering events called "allostasis," result in an effort by the body to regain balance, or "homeostasis." This homeostasis, while ensuring cellular function and species survival in the short term, might not feel definitively well to the patient. Insulin resistance, as an example, in the individual with chronically high blood sugar, is an adaptive state. High levels of glucose inside the cell form advanced glycation end-products with cellular components like proteins, lipids, and even DNA, and wreak molecular havoc. As blood sugar levels continue to climb, it takes more insulin from the pancreas to achieve blood sugar balance, and all the while, tissue insulin resistance is attempting to protect the inside of the cell. When allostatic overload is reached, the scale tips, and diabetes becomes the new norm. The body remains in this state, perpetuated by the factors that keep it on the same trajectory. We can bring hope for a patient and the possibility of achieving-re-balance, or health once again, but we must first enable ourselves to recognize those triggering events. We must open our eyes to those smaller but significant perturbations and factors that lead to overload of the system in the first place, as well as those which mediate the pattern of illness. Then we can identify the new path that will lead to restoration.

Here are the seven functional biological systems:

ASSIMILATION

We begin with Assimilation, which is primarily represented by the gut. We are going to spend a lot of time here. Assimilation refers to the process of digesting or absorbing nutrients. While this is a function of the digestive tract, it also includes the lungs, where we respire oxygen, and the skin, which is capable of absorbing nutrients and chemicals, and excreting waste through its surface.

Digestion begins in the mouth, where the process of mastication, or the chewing of food, is the start of the process of breaking down food into smaller particulate matter that can be more easily processed. Food is mixed with salivary enzymes, and it is the first place of physical contact, where food begins its interaction with the central nervous system through touch, taste, smell, and the movement of the tongue and jaw. The nerve signals herald the release of digestive juices and hormones as food enters the stomach through the lower esophageal sphincter. Gastric acid helps to break down the smaller protein chunks, and provides the appropriate environment for the absorption of key nutrients such as vitamin B12, iron, calcium, and magnesium.

This process continues in the small intestines, where the pulpy, acidic fluid called chyme is further processed by the enzymes secreted by the pancreas, and bile that has been produced by the liver is released from its holding area, the gallbladder. In the intact small intestine, nutrients are transported across the one-cell-thick layer known as the epithelium. It is a remarkable feat. Through the coordinated efforts of the resident immune system in the gut, and the microbes which make their home in that part of the intestine, nutrients can be separated and identified from non-digestible matter and absorbed. The remainder passes further down the digestive tract to eventually be excreted.

The large intestine, or colon, plays a critical role in the absorption of water from the digested matter. It is the home for the majority of intestinal microflora that play a critical role in breaking down substances from the chyme that have not been digested so far. As a result, these microbes produce several critical vitamins in the B family, as well as vitamin K, and short-chain fatty acids such as butyrate, both of which play key roles in energy metabolism in the brain.

The production of these short-chain fatty acids comes from the consumption of insoluble fiber in our diet. The microbes that inhabit the digestive tract, from the mouth to the anus, perform a multitude of key biological functions in the human body. They give rise to the idea that we are in fact an ecosystem, living symbiotically with our microbial brethren. Like the ecosystems that are part of our external world, imbalances within this ecosystem can lead to substantial disruptions in function and vitality. It should not come as a surprise that disruptions of the human microbial ecosystem have been associated with a wide variety of diseases, including those that affect the brain, such as Alzheimer's disease, multiple sclerosis, Parkinson's disease, and amyotrophic lateral sclerosis. These disruptions are characterized by not only changes in the overall microbial diversity of the gut microbiome, but also the balance of individual organisms. For example, in one study of stool composition taken from participants with Alzheimer's disease, compared to the control group, those affected had decreased *Firmicutes*, increased *Bacteroidetes*, and decreased *Bifidobacterium*[15]. In multiple sclerosis, one group of researchers identified specific bacteria that were significantly associated the disease, *Akkermansia muciniphila* and *Acinetobacter calcoaceticus*. These bacteria produced an inflammatory response in human white blood cells. In contrast, *Parabacteroides distasonis*, which was reduced in MS patients, stimulated an anti-inflammatory response[16]. In a mouse model of Amyotrophic Lateral Sclerosis, a shifted profile of the intestinal microbiome, including reduced levels of *Butyrivibrio Fibrisolvens*, *Escherichia coli*, and *Fermicus*[17].

Going beyond this critically important subject of the gut microbiome and its relation to brain disease, it is necessary to think of the digestive system as a whole. The basic question as to the adequacy and quality of food intake needs to be considered. Has there been sufficient consumption of foods rich in B-vitamins, antioxidant vitamins E and C, the anti-inflammatory omega-3 fatty acids? Is there an appropriate gut environment for breaking down whole foods, specifically, adequate production of digestive enzymes and levels of hydrochloric acid in the stomach? What is the status of bile production which aids in the emulsification and absorption of fats, including fat-soluble vitamins, like A, D, and E? Is there sufficient insoluble fiber intake for production of the short-chain fatty acids (which takes place in the colon, as mentioned earlier)? How do conditions like chronic constipation affect the body's ability to eliminate toxins? Moreover, when these imbalances do occur, how do they affect the other functional biological systems, including the energy-producing factories of the cell, the mitochondria, and the immune system?

Before we leave the system of Assimilation, there is one other area to explore, and that is the connection between the gut and the brain. This is a bidirectional system of communication where signals from the digestive tract alter the function and health of the brain, and the brain, in turn, sends signals to the gut to alter its behavior. For the purpose of our discussion, I am going to focus mainly on the ways in which the digestive system sends signals to the brain. I have already presented two examples in which alterations in the gut microbial community have pro- or anti-inflammatory effects and modulate the risk of diseases, like Alzheimer's and multiple sclerosis. The information database continues to grow, with respect to the relationship between gut microbiota and neurological diseases. Parkinson's disease is another example and serves as a model to discuss this gut-brain connection. Here, evidence suggests, like with the other conditions, that a pro-inflammatory microbial profile is present, with increased abundance of *Enterobacteriaceae*, and lower abundance of *Prevotella* and other short-chain fatty acid-producing bacteria[18]. *Prevotella* are also promoters of thiamine and folate synthesis, and these nutrients have been found in lower levels in Parkinson's patients[19].

Two other key features of the gut connection to the brain are exemplified in Parkinson's disease. The vagus nerve is one of 12 cranial nerves that send their signals to the brain or receive signals from the brain primarily for functions of the head (such as smell, sight, eye movement, facial sensation and movement, tongue movement, and taste). It also has a much larger role to play in the body. Nicknamed "the wanderer" from its Latin derivation, the vagus nerve sends and receives signals from numerous parts of the body and viscera, including the larynx or vocal cords, heart, lungs, and digestive tract. In the gut, signals from the vagus nerve are involved in acid release in the stomach, normal gut motility, secretion of digestive enzymes, influence over the immune response, and gut barrier function. In turn, the vagus nerve sends information to the brain about nutrient availability, absorption, eating behavior, and satiety. In Parkinson's disease, the direct connection between the gut and brain via the vagus nerve appears to be a key player in the initiation and progression of the disease. Chronic constipation, likely due to multiple factors including gut motility, is recognized as an important pre-clinical predictor of Parkinson's disease. Moreover, the vagus nerve is a transit route for the hallmark pathological finding in the brains of those with Parkinson's disease. The abnormal protein called alpha-synuclein, toxic to brain cells, appears to be formed in the gut where the microbiome plays a major role in its production[20].

The last important connection between the gut and brain to be discussed is that of the gut wall itself. The intestinal tissue lining is known as the epithelium, and the cells are called enterocytes. The barrier between the inside lumen of the gut (the location of the chyme, digestive juices, hormones, microbes, and immune cells) is separated from the bloodstream by this layer of tissue that is one enterocyte cell thick. The intestinal epithelium acts as a selective barrier to prevent the entry of harmful substances into the blood, while allowing the entry of nutrients, electrolytes, and water. This feat is accomplished in part by the architecture of the intestinal epithelium, which, as a result of specialized transport proteins, allows some of substances to pass directly through the cells themselves, such as amino acids, fatty acids, sugars, vitamins, and minerals. This transcellular movement is accomplished by specialized transport proteins. An alternate mode of transport is when substances travel through spaces between the intestinal epithelial cells. Normally, this is limited to water and electrolytes[21]. These spaces are known as tight junctions, and a protein called zonulin plays a major role in regulating the permeability of this barrier[22]. The phenomenon in which this selective gut barrier becomes disrupted is known as "increased gut permeability," or by the more common term, "leaky gut." A whole host of factors within each of the functional biological systems plays a role in driving inflammation and oxidative stress in the gut, thereby triggering

"Leaky Gut Syndrome." These factors include imbalances in the gut microbial community, immune response, hormones, blood supply, toxin exposure, alterations in cellular energy production, and failure of antioxidant defense mechanisms. For this reason, management of leaky gut is often considered the focal point of a functional medicine strategy to manage chronic disease. Heal the gut, and you can come a long way toward healing the brain.

The gut is also the home for part of our system of defense and repair, where it serves as a protective interface between the outer world and our internal world. This is called the gut-associated lymphoid tissue, and it is an important component of the immune system as a whole. This will be discussed further in Defense & Repair.

DEFENSE & REPAIR

Defense & Repair is the second node among the biological systems, where clinical imbalances can lead to illness or disease. It is a major component of that process reviewed earlier, inflammation. The coordinated efforts of a variety of white blood cell types, signaling molecules called cytokines, and bioactive nutrients such as omega-3 and omega-6 fatty acids stored in the cell membranes, play key roles in our protection and the repair of damaged tissue.

Bear in mind that the main role for the immune system is to be able to recognize things that are "not self," foreign, or pose a threat to your health. These immune triggers are sometimes referred to as antigens. There are two key responses to antigens, and they involve what is referred to as humoral and cellular immunity. Specific white blood cell types are involved in these different responses. The humoral immune response, also called the antibody-mediated immune response, triggers white blood cells known as B cells to develop into plasma cells and secrete large amounts of antibodies. These antibodies target the perceived foreign invader directly or indirectly, to orchestrate its demise. Viruses typically trigger an antibody response, and we can gauge prior exposure and immunity to those viruses by evaluating blood for viral antibodies.

Cellular immunity, also called the cell-mediated immune response, is an immune response by white blood cells known as T-cells, which in turn activate and direct other immune cells, such as macrophages, to destroy infected cells or pathogens. Some T-cells mature into so called "T-killer cells," capable of directly recognizing and destroying cancer cells or cells infected by viruses.

It is important to remember that the immune system also plays a role in tissue repair. The immune system cells secrete several cytokines, growth factors, and enzymes, which promote not only the resolution of inflammation, but repair and regeneration. In some cases, that tissue repair may result in scar formation or fibrosis, and in others, the tissue repair includes the promotion of signaling molecules that lead to the growth of new blood vessels necessary to maintaining the health of the regenerated tissue.

We can reframe our thinking about the behavior of our systems of Defense & Repair when we consider the concept of homeostasis mentioned earlier. Here, balance means an immune system that is neither underactive nor overactive. An underactive immune system can lead to chronic infection, and an overactive immune system may lead to autoimmunity, a condition in which the immune system is unable to regulate itself, and attacks our own body tissues as if they were foreign.

Infectious mechanisms have been implicated in a variety of neurological diseases. Several have been associated with the risk of Alzheimer's disease. For example, Herpes Simplex Virus-1, and bacteria including *Chlamydia pneumoniae*, *Helicobacter pylori*, and the Lyme disease-causing *Borrelia burgdorferi*[23]. Infectious triggers for multiple sclerosis supported by research include Human Herpes Virus-6, Epstein Barr Virus, and *Chlamydia pneumonia*[24]. An interesting development is the potentially protective role that helminths (parasites *Trypanosoma cruzi* and *Paracoccidioides brasiliensis*) might play in regulating the behavior of the immune system in diseases like MS. One study examined blood markers of patients with MS who were infected with the helminths and compared them to controls. The investigators found that those infected had higher levels of brain-derived neurotrophic factor, nerve growth factor, and B-cell-derived IL-10 (an anti-inflammatory cytokine)[25]. It appears that these parasite infections actually confer a protective effect (by the way, also a gut-brain connection). This invokes the idea that our hygiene-obsessed culture, by lowering the risk of helminth infections through water sanitation, may actually create an imbalance in the immune system, thereby increasing susceptibility to autoimmunity.

Autoimmunity occurs in a genetically susceptible individual whose immune system is challenged by some environmental trigger, such as tissue injury or infection. The immune system regulates its behavior through a variety of signals, including the balance between proinflammatory (such as Interleukin-1β, Interleukin-6, and Tumor Necrosis Factor-α) and anti-inflammatory cytokines (such as Interleukin-10 and Transforming Growth Factor-β), and the role that regulatory T-cells play to counterbalance attack-positioned cytotoxic T-killer cells. However, in autoimmunity, this balance has been disrupted, leading to defective tolerance or regulation, meaning the degree to which the immune system can ignore the self and not see it as foreign. This can be due to increased and persistent presence of tissue that is normally cleared or alteration in that tissue, for example, from injury, in such a way that the immune system sees it as "not self" or potentially threatening. In some cases, viral or bacterial infections may contribute to autoimmunity by triggering the activation of T-cells that cross-react with self-antigens in a phenomenon known as molecular mimicry. Among the conditions discussed in this book, multiple sclerosis is most characteristically autoimmune in nature. However, whereas inflammation plays a role in all of the chronic conditions affecting the brain, the goal of functional medicine is to rein in the activity of the immune system. It achieves this goal by identifying the underlying environmental triggers, correcting the imbalances, and nurturing a shift (through innate homeostatic mechanisms) that reflects a set point of healthy immune balance.

There are a few other key concepts when it comes to understanding this Defense & Repair system, in relationship to the brain. The first is the blood-brain barrier. This is a highly selective defensive wall, of sorts. It exists at the interface between the cells that line the blood vessels in the brain and the neural tissues themselves, both neurons and support cells. Its function is to allow for the movement of water, glucose, amino acids, hormones, oxygen, carbon dioxide, and some lipid-soluble molecules into the brain itself, while restricting entry of other molecules, potential toxins and infectious agents. An intact blood-brain barrier is critical for brain health and brain immune system balance. But inflammatory drivers affect the leakiness or permeability of this barrier.

In the last section, the topic of leaky gut was discussed. Compromise of the gut barrier can lead to release of pro-inflammatory toxins into the blood, known as lipid-polysaccharides (LPS). These are the outer membranes of gram negative bacteria, such as *Escherichia coli*. LPS is a major driver of inflammation and disease affecting the brain. In the Alzheimer's susceptible brain, LPS causes buildup of the protein beta amyloid-42, which, in turn, leads to loss of synaptic connection between brain cells and decline in cognitive function[26]. The same mechanism has been demonstrated in an experimental model of multiple sclerosis[27], in Parkinson's disease[28], and in the blood of patients with sporadic amyotrophic lateral sclerosis[29]. Thus, there is a parallel between the selectively permeable barrier of the endothelial gut wall and the blood stream, and the endothelial-lined vascular wall of the blood-brain barrier. Each has its own associated immune system. The gut has the gut-associated lymphoid tissue and the brain has the microglia. The peripheral immune system cells can more easily penetrate the brain as well, when the blood-brain barrier has been compromised.

A second component worth touching upon is nuclear factor kappa-light-chain-enhancer of activated B cells, or NF-kB. This is a protein complex stored in the liquid component of the inside of cells in the inactive state, until called upon for its powerful properties. In the brain, NF-kB can be found in the microglia and nerve cell support cells known as astrocytes. When activated, NF-kB travels to the center of the cell known as the nucleus, the location of the DNA, where it activates elements leading to the transcription of proteins involved in the immune response. The activation of NF-kB is under tight control within the cell, but serves diverse functions in the nervous system (including learning and memory) by influencing the connections between nerve cells. At the same time, dysregulation of NF-kB has been linked to aging, and to degenerative and inflammatory diseases of the nervous system[30].

A noteworthy transition from Defense & Repair into Biotransformation & Elimination, and Transport, is a discussion of the recently discovered waste clearance system from the brain known as the glymphatic system. Outside of the brain, the lymphatic system has a parallel function and can be seen as part of the immune system and part of the body's system for elimination of waste products and cellular debris. The name "glymphatic" comes from the glial cells, which comprise the family of support cells for neurons (nerve cells) within the brain and spinal cord. Glial cells include: the **microglia**, which are the immune cells of the brain; **astrocytes**, which provide structural and metabolic support; **oligodendrocytes**, which form the fatty nerve sheath known as "myelin," and enhance electrical conduction; and **ependymal** cells, which play a role in the production of spinal fluid. The glymphatic system promotes elimination of soluble proteins and metabolites from the central nervous system and helps distribute non-waste compounds such as glucose, lipids, amino acids, and neurotransmitters. (Neurotransmitters are the chemical signals secreted by nerve cells that allow them to communicate with one another.) The glymphatic system, primarily active during sleep, forms another important connection between the brain and the rest of the body. Impairment of normal glymphatic flow from the brain has been implicated in the literature as an important mechanism, when it comes to understanding the chronic effects of traumatic brain injury[31], the aging brain[32], and Alzheimer's disease[33]. In basic terms, insufficient or poor-quality sleep results in impaired clearance of toxins from the brain, and contributes to brain inflammation. This underlies the fact that sleep serves many critical functions beyond the restoration of wakefulness following a good night of sleep.

BIOTRANSFORMATION & ELIMINATION and TRANSPORT

Biotransformation & Elimination and Transport refer to how the body handles waste, and the means by which it transports waste, cells, nutrients, gases, and electrolytes. This latter system of Transport includes the blood vessels, lymphatics, and the glymphatics. Waste can be defined as the by-products of cellular reactions that require elimination by the body (such as ammonia – a product of protein metabolism), indigestible foodstuffs, dead cells and other detritus, and environmental toxins that have found their way into the body and must be eliminated. Many toxins are found in nature, such as arsenic in soil. Our modern industrial age has introduced additional toxins into our environment at a rate and magnitude many times greater than our biological waste removal systems have evolved to handle. In a sense, life in modern times has put these waste management systems on double duty because they are the same systems necessary for eliminating toxins our bodies produce and would encounter in nature, but they are called upon to eliminate industrial, commercial chemical and pharmaceutical waste, as well. These systems are found in every cell, but are concentrated in organs such as the liver and kidneys. Fundamentally, the way the body gets rid of toxins is through a two-step process.

The first step of elimination involves a family of enzymes known as cytochrome P450. The product of this step is then conjugated, or connected to another molecule, to make that product more water soluble. The product of this second step can then be excreted. Sometimes the cytochrome P450-metabolized product is also toxic, such as when benzo[a]pyrene found in coal tar, tobacco smoke, and grilled foods is converted to its intermediate metabolite[34], a carcinogenic compound linked to lung and colon cancer.

Toxic overload, therefore, can occur either because of the magnitude of the exposure, the products formed from the metabolism of these compounds, or impairment in the body's ability to excrete the toxin. Not only is our waste excreted through the stool and kidneys (shedding light on the importance of regular bowel movements and adequate hydration for kidney function), but also through the skin and lungs. Furthermore, one of the body's key antioxidants, glutathione, is also one of the compounds used in these conjugation reactions. Toxins, therefore, that put a large demand on the body's supply of glutathione, limit its availability as an antioxidant and for other elimination reactions. A deficit of glutathione can lead to mitochondrial failure, organ failure, or death. A classic example is acetaminophen-induced liver toxicity. In the United States, it accounts for more than 50% of overdose-related acute liver failure cases and approximately 20% of the liver transplant cases[35].

Several toxins can harm the brain and increase the risk of cognitive decline and dementia. These include lead, mercury, aluminum, arsenic, high levels of manganese, and a variety of pesticides, flame retardants, solvents, air pollutants, plasticizers, and certain drugs, such as anesthetic agents[36]. Besides exposure, the operative concept is "bioaccumulation," or how much of these toxins accumulate in the body, over time. In part, this is dependent upon how readily the toxin is stored (such as in fat tissue), and the capability of the body to eliminate the toxin rapidly and effectively. Not all toxins are heavy metals or chemicals. Biological toxins or "biotoxins" are produced by living organisms. The disease botulism can be considered a biotoxin illness because *botulinum* toxin is produced by a bacterium known as *Clostridium botulinum*. It causes death through its effect as a neuromuscular blocking agent, leading to respiratory failure. More insidious are the mycotoxins produced by molds found in water-damaged buildings, which can cause neurological and psychiatric symptoms by dysregulating pathways that control inflammatory signaling[37].

A story that touched my life in 1990 serves as an example of how chemical exposure and biotransformation can lead to the production of a toxin capable of mimicking a familiar disease of the brain. I was about halfway through my four-year medical school degree at Emory University when the department of neurology brought in a new chairman named Mahlon Delong. Dr. Delong still practices, teaches, and does research at Emory. He arrived in Atlanta accompanied by several of his colleagues from Johns Hopkins University in Baltimore, where they were making a significant impact on neuroscience research in the area of Parkinson's disease. Emory had a lot to offer Dr. Delong and his team, particularly the availability of the Yerkes Primate Research Center on campus. Dr. Delong's work involved a model of Parkinson's disease that had been set in motion by an accident about eight years earlier, in Northern California. The discovery began with the hospitalization of a patient at the Santa Clara Valley Medical Center in San Jose, a teaching hospital associated with Stanford University[38]. There, a male drug addict was admitted to the psychiatric unit with an unusual presentation thought initially to be a case of catatonic schizophrenia. In this form of schizophrenia, the patient appears to be awake but is immobile and otherwise unresponsive. Upon closer examination, he had features strikingly similar to Parkinson's disease. Eventually, seven other addicts were identified and the spectrum of their physical findings included rest tremor, lead pipe-like rigidity of muscle tone, and a cog-wheeling sensation felt by the examiner when the arm is passively moved. Nearly all responded to the treatment commonly used in Parkinson's disease, the drug Levodopa. It turned out that these seven individuals had accidentally injected a form of synthetic heroin found to contain large quantities of a compound known as MPTP. MPTP or 1-methyl-4-phenly-1,2,3,6-tetrahydrapyridine is formed when another compound, called MPPP, similar to the narcotic meperidine, is being made, but what they injected was nearly pure MPTP.

Not only did the drug addicts appear to acquire Parkinson's disease after exposure to this toxic compound, but examination of the brain of one of them who died revealed that the same area of the brain affected in Parkinson's was also affected in these cases.

Furthermore, it was determined that when MPTP is metabolized in the body, it is transformed to a compound called MPP+, and MPP+ is toxic to the energy producing factories of the cell — the mitochondria. Out of the tragedy of these original seven heroin addicts who developed a syndrome nearly identical to Parkinson's disease came a body of research aimed at further understanding of what causes this debilitating illness, the role of the mitochondria, and treatment options that would help those affected by it.

Dr. Delong and his colleagues studied the MPTP model with chimpanzees, and their research led to the development of an approach now in clinical use, called Deep Brain Stimulation (DBS). It has helped individuals around the world who suffer from advanced Parkinson's. In DBS, wires are implanted in the brain, where they deliver electrical pulses to significantly reduce the disabling symptoms. The research has also broadened our understanding of how damage to mitochondria contributes to neuroinflammatory and neurodegenerative diseases.

ENERGY

This discussion of mitochondria brings us to the next node among the functional biological systems, referred to as Energy. We are living beings, and life requires energy at every moment of our existence. The energy that drives cellular biochemistry is called adenosine triphosphate, and the factories that produce this energy are mitochondria. "Tri-" phosphate refers to three phosphate groups. Each of these phosphates forms a high energy bond on a backbone consisting of the nucleic acid adenine and the 5-carbon sugar ribose. When the bond is broken, its energy is released. Mitochondria are more numerous in tissues like brain, heart, and skeletal muscle because these tissues demand so much energy. Examine an individual cell, and you will find them floating in the cell's watery inner substance, known as the cytosol.

Mitochondria are able to use nutrients from our diet (carbohydrates in the form of glucose, fats, and if necessary, protein) to produce these high-energy molecules. When a phosphate bond is broken, the energy stored in that bond is released. The optimal production of ATP requires oxygen, and the products of this process, aside from ATP, are carbon dioxide and water. Glucose and fat are the primary sources of fuel for the mitochondria, with fat being used during times of fasting, while glucose is utilized more disproportionately during periods of high intensity movement or exercise.

Several nutrient cofactors are required for the efficient metabolism of fats and glucose into ATP. These include magnesium, carnitine, lipoic acid, B vitamins (B1, B2, B3), iron, manganese, and glutathione. Like MPP+, several toxic metals can impair mitochondrial function, including arsenic, mercury, aluminum, antimony, and the trace mineral fluoride. The use of oxygen by mitochondria to create adenosine triphosphate normally results in the production of pro-oxidant reactive oxygen species. To protect mitochondria, glutathione, the cell's main antioxidant defense, must be present in sufficient supply. Not surprisingly, high levels of oxidative stress act as a signal to the cell to synthesize more glutathione. Low levels of mitochondrial glutathione are associated with Parkinson's disease, multiple sclerosis, and the amyloid beta-induced inflammation that contributes to Alzheimer's disease. Among the nutrient factors that play a direct or indirect role in the synthesis of glutathione are the vitamins folate and B12, the amino acid cysteine, and alpha lipoic acid. Vitamins C and E also protect mitochondria by acting as antioxidants.

Perhaps the biggest counter to the effects of inflammation and oxidative stress, including those directed by NF-kB activation is another nuclear regulatory factor known as Nuclear factor erythroid 2-related factor or Nrf2, for short. Nrf2 has emerged as a key player in the cellular dance where inflammatory and oxidative stress signals are counterbalanced by anti-inflammatory and antioxidant elements. It is a protein that can be activated inside of every cell which, when called upon, directs the DNA within the cell's nucleus to increase the production of antioxidant enzymes such as catalase, superoxide dismutase, and glutathione. Nrf2 thereby protects mitochondria against excessive oxidative stress, while facilitating cellular detoxification.

COMMUNICATION

As we move along the interconnected nodes of the functional biological systems, next is Communication. Communication refers to the ways in which different types of cells throughout the body are able to talk to one another, transfer information, and ultimately create biological responses. The chemicals involved in cellular communication include hormones (otherwise known as the endocrine system), neurotransmitters (the chemical signals that allow one nerve cell to communicate with another), and the immune messengers we have already discussed, known as cytokines.

A simple rule of thumb is that glands, which produce and secrete hormones, communicate their information across large distances, generally throughout the body, via the bloodstream, to multiple tissues, both outside and inside (or across) the blood-brain barrier. Neurotransmitters, secreted primarily for nerve to nerve communication or nerve to muscle communication, travel a short distance across what is known as the synaptic cleft. In the brain, the long arms of nerve cells known as axons end in a region known as the synaptic bouton. Here, the neurotransmitters are stored in small spheres called synaptic vesicles, ready to be released by the cell.

At the other side of the synaptic cleft, the postsynaptic neuron (which has sprouted long spines known as dendrites from its cell body), receives the chemical information when the neurotransmitter binds to a protein receptor on the surface of the dendrite. This may trigger an electrical impulse known as an action potential. However, some signals coming from presynaptic nerve cells are actually inhibitory, rather than excitatory, and make it less likely that the postsynaptic nerve cell or neuron will generate its electrical signal.

The classic excitatory neurotransmitter is glutamate, and there is a variety of glutamate receptor subtypes. GABA, or gamma-aminobutyric acid, is the main inhibitory neurotransmitter in the human brain. The synthesis of neurotransmitters requires an adequate supply of the amino acids tyrosine, tryptophan, glutamic acid, the vitamin choline, and B vitamins such as folate and B12. Here is a recurring theme — that food, besides the pleasure it brings and our sense of satiety, is information for the brain. The availability of choline — found in meat, poultry, fish, and eggs — affects the synthesis of acetylcholine stored in the nerve cells of the hippocampus (a region on the inside surface of the brain's temporal lobe involved in short-term memory and classically affected in Alzheimer's disease). Glutamate receptors are distributed more widely throughout the brain, and glutamate plays a major role in memory and learning. GABA, serotonin, norepinephrine, and acetylcholine each play a role in sleep, whereas serotonin and norepinephrine also play roles in attentiveness and emotion. While glutamate is the most important neurotransmitter involved in learning, all neurotransmitters have been identified as having roles to play in this process.

The function of hormones, from growth to reproduction, to feeding and satiety, to energy storage and release, to metabolism, connects them to the node of Communication. For the purposes of this book, the main hormones of interest include cortisol, progesterone, testosterone, estrogen, thyroid hormone, insulin, and melatonin.

Cortisol is synthesized in the adrenal glands, which sit on top of the kidneys on the right and left sides of the body. It is made from cholesterol, as are the other hormones that broadly fall under the umbrella of gonadal hormones (including progesterone, testosterone, and the estrogens: estriol, estradiol, and estrone). Another hormone produced from cholesterol is aldosterone, which is responsible for helping maintain fluid balance through its regulation of sodium and potassium levels in the body.

The release of cortisol from the adrenal glands under normal conditions follows a pattern that repeats itself every 24 hours. Cortisol rises in the early morning hours, then gradually drops over the course of the day. As a protective hormone, it prepares and protects our bodies from the stressors we may encounter, especially while awake. It helps regulate blood sugar levels. Like aldosterone, it plays a role in sodium and potassium balance. It subdues the behavior of the immune system broadly and deeply by not only suppressing T-cells, for example, but the protein signal NF-kB that acts as an "on" switch to signal DNA transcription of a range of proinflammatory cytokines. I like to think of NF-kB as the main circuit breaker in the electrical box in your home.

Recall that inflammation is involved in tissue repair, an energy-dependent process that takes place during sleep. But the period of wakefulness is one that necessarily demands increased vigilance (cortisol), particularly for our hunter-gatherer ancestors, with whom we are nearly identical genetically, despite our modern ways. Protection trumps tissue repair for the hunter and the hunted.

The hippocampus of the brain is dense with cortisol receptors. This observation brings together the roles of stress and fear with learning and memory. In the short term, stress and fear may reinforce and therefore benefit learning and memory. But when the brain, especially the hippocampus, is chronically exposed to this hormone, it can have detrimental effects.

The release of cortisol is under the command of two adjacent structures in the brain, the pituitary gland and the hypothalamus. Survival is our most primitive instinct and arguably our prime biological directive, so that we may reproduce and pass on our genetic material. The brain will send adaptive, homeostatic signals to the adrenal glands after a period of time that cortisol secretion has been excessive and prolonged, and will eventually suppress the production of cortisol. There are many consequences to this cortisol suppression, including its impact on memory, pain, tissue repair, strength, energy, and mood. This should seem familiar to those suffering from conditions like Chronic Fatigue and Fibromyalgia[39].

Although progesterone plays a specific role in human reproduction by helping the uterus to prepare for implantation and to maintain pregnancy once it has occurred, it plays a separate role in the brain. In the central nervous system, progesterone affects the excitability of neurons and their support cells, the glia. Through its action on GABA receptors, progesterone exerts a calming, even sedating, anti-anxiety effect. To an extent, it counters the excitatory effect of cortisol and promotes tissue repair by stimulating the formation of myelin, the fatty protective coating around nerve cell axons that facilitates signal transmission at high speeds.

While both testosterone and estrogen play key roles in the sexual and reproductive characteristics of men and women, they also play important roles in the brain. These hormones affect learning and mood, and estrogen in particular seems to have an effect on the risk of developing Alzheimer's disease later in life. Testosterone appears to have some protective benefit, as well. Approximately ⅔ of older Americans living with Alzheimer's disease are women. The Cache County Study on Memory and Aging (a large, population-based study started in 1995) found that women who used any form of hormone replacement therapy within five years of menopause had a 30 percent reduced risk of Alzheimer's disease, particularly when taken for 10 or more years[40]. The Mayo Clinic Cohort Study of Oophorectomy and Aging showed that women whose ovaries were surgically removed before the age of 45 had about a 5-fold increased risk of mortality from neurological or mental disease, including parkinsonism, cognitive impairment and dementia, depression, and anxiety[41]. However, this risk could be mitigated in women who started hormone replacement therapy after oophorectomy and continued treatment until at least the natural age of menopause. Interestingly, results of the Women's Health Initiative suggested that women who initiated estrogen therapy alone or in combination with a progestin later in life, 65-79 years, experienced an *increased* risk of dementia and cognitive decline, regardless of the type of menopause[42]. There appears to be a window of opportunity for hormone replacement to be initiated early to protect a woman's aging brain.

Thyroid hormone has an impact on brain development and function throughout life. Low thyroid hormone, called hypothyroidism, during the neonatal period, is known to have long-lasting effects on behavior and performance through structural brain alteration, decreased myelination, and alterations in nerve cell maturation. In the adult brain, thyroid hormone has effects on mood and behavior by altering the sensitivity of serotonin receptors. Hypothyroidism can be an underlying cause of dementia. Interestingly, the autoimmune disorder known as Hashimoto's thyroiditis, in which antibodies to thyroid peroxidase are produced, can not only lead to symptoms of hypothyroidism such as dry skin, hair loss, constipation, joint stiffness, and muscle weakness, but it can also affect the brain. The antibodies are associated with a condition of altered awareness known as Hashimoto's encephalopathy. Individuals with this condition can present with a wide spectrum of neurological symptoms that can include confusion, tremor, speech problems, and even seizures, whereas normal function of thyroid hormone on the brain exerts a near opposite effect. However, it should be pointed out that the mechanisms of Hashimoto's encephalopathy on the brain, while inflammatory, do not appear to be a direct antibody effect[43]. Chronically elevated levels of cortisol will decrease the levels of the signaling hormone, Thyroid Stimulating Hormone, secreted by the pituitary gland, thereby lowering thyroid hormone production. It also inhibits the conversion of two forms of thyroid hormone, thyroxine (T4, secreted by the thyroid gland) into triiodothyronine (T3, mainly produced at the tissue level). Furthermore, these same chronically elevated levels of cortisol can inhibit reproduction through their effect on the hypothalamus and pituitary glands, which normally signal the testes and ovaries, by influencing the pathway that produces progesterone, testosterone, and estrogen.

Insulin, a hormone secreted by the pancreas, which plays a major role in glucose metabolism, affects the brain through its influence on feeding behavior, and plays a role in the brain's oversight of energy stores. But insulin is important in memory and learning. When cells become resistant to the effect of insulin, which normally facilitates the transport of glucose from the blood into the cells, the result is an impaired ability to store immediate and remote memory, and it contributes to the risk of Alzheimer's disease[44].

Finally, melatonin, a hormone released by the pineal gland in the brain and produced from serotonin, is important for its role in synchronizing the circadian clock and letting us know when it is time to go to sleep. Like other hormones, melatonin appears to have multiple functions, including its role as an antioxidant and anti-inflammatory molecule.

STRUCTURAL INTEGRITY

The clinical node that is Structural Integrity, the last node to be explored, binds all the other nodes together. Structural Integrity can refer to the musculoskeletal structure that gives us our shape or form, and allows us to move as a bipedal species on earth. Imbalances in musculoskeletal control, such as awkward, persistent, or sustained alterations in posture, movement, and mobility can result in injury to the joints and spine. It also references structure at the tissue level, such as the gut-circulation interface or the blood-brain barrier, the individual cell membrane, and subcellular membranes. The fatty phospholipid bilayer that makes up the structure of cell walls is dependent upon the balance of dietary omega-3 and omega-6 polyunsaturated fatty acids, suggesting that dietary deficiency of these essential nutrients can profoundly alter structure and function, all the way down to the level of the cell. Structural integrity can refer to the integrity of the DNA or RNA strands (**D**eoxyribo**N**ucleic **A**cid and **R**ibo**N**ucleic **A**cid) which contain the information we refer to as the "code of life." Disruptions of nucleic acid integrity are associated with cancers, cell death from radiation exposure, and toxin exposure, and almost always involve inflammation and oxidative stress as an intermediary process, en route to disease and death.

It is apparent in this discussion that each node has a broad range of functions that affects multiple systems. No one system dominates and no one system acts entirely separately from the others. In my office, I sometimes refer to the image of a Ferris wheel, and ask my patients to remember that in this wonder of mechanical engineering, no one car is on top at all times. The wheel is in constant motion. This idea that everything affects everything, and everything is interconnected forms the basis for functional medicine and the framework for a therapeutic approach that is truly holistic. It is no wonder that the targeted therapeutic approaches of drugs cannot possibly address all the imbalances within the systems that contribute to disease, and why conventional treatment never results in a return to health. It is not possible to entirely separate one functional system from the others. It makes even less sense, you should now understand, to engage in a dialogue about treating illness by a singular organ system, as well.

CHAPTER 6

The Clues are in the History

How Your Story Can Help You Learn What You Need to Do to Protect Your Brain

"When we talk about understanding, surely it takes place only when the mind listens completely — the mind being your heart, your nerves, your ears — when you give your whole attention to it."

—Jiddu Krishnamurti, philosopher and teacher

Many years ago, Dr. Stone told me that the link between the narrative in literature and medicine was the patient history. While on rounds in the hospital visiting his sick patients, the story that each one would share with him was a potent opportunity for the writer to build his scrapbook of ideas from the riches of human experience. "I would go into the hospital room, and gently take Jane's arm by the wrist, feeling for her radial pulse, make contact through touch. I would ask her how she was doing? She would tell me, and it would be a story." Thirty years ago, as a student, I too learned the nuts and bolts of gathering the medical history from my patients. While a useful and, in fact, critical tool for diagnosis in conventional medicine, the current structure of the medical history as it is obtained by the physician does not easily lend itself to understanding disease from the root cause perspective. The technique is guided by specific questions and experiences.

Let's review what happens in a doctor's office. You arrive and fill out forms indicating your medications, allergies, any conditions for which you are being treated, and check a long list of symptoms or health problems you may have known as the "review of systems." Your vital signs are obtained and entered into a computer, along with the other information you have provided. Primarily, the time spent on history with the doctor is focused on the "History of Present Illness," the main problem or concern you wish to discuss or have evaluated. This narrative progresses by covering specific key points, such as location, quality, severity, duration, timing, things that make it worse or better, and additional associated symptoms.

Here is an example. Barbie is a 42 year old woman who started having disabling headaches when she was 14 years old. The headaches began shortly after her first menstrual period. Over the years, they became more frequent, now about four times per month. Although sometimes they come with onset of her menses, this is not always the case. She can wake up with a headache, but it may occur later in the day. The pain progresses over an hour or two before it is maximal. The right side of the head is involved, especially above the right eye and around the right temple. The pain is throbbing or pulsating in quality. She becomes nauseated and sometimes vomits. There is light and sound sensitivity. Activity, such as climbing stairs, will make her symptoms worse. She goes into a dark, quiet room, and lies down with a cool cloth over her head. The symptoms will last all day, or until she goes to sleep.

Her past medical and surgical history, personal life history and habits, allergies, and family health history — though important — are not given as much weight in the diagnostic puzzle as the history of present illness.

Barbie has a normal physical examination.

She is diagnosed with migraine, and she is offered treatment. It is possible that her treatment might include a plan for stress reduction, avoidance of certain foods, or an attempt to improve her sleep quality. Generally, however, the visit will end with a recommendation of medication that can help stop her migraines when they occur, and prevent as many as possible from occurring in the first place. In this strategy the information is organized in such a way as to bring both physician and patient to a conclusion about a diagnosis, then match a treatment plan to the diagnosis. In other words, it is the "pill for an ill" approach.

By contrast, the timeline of a person's life, from their past family history to their prenatal and birth periods, through events of childhood and adulthood, all of that medical, surgical, and social history, allergies, and family history, is the perfect approach to explore illness in functional medicine. There is an expression that says "Genes load the gun, but environment pulls the trigger," and in order to understand how a person got sick, it is necessary to explore the complete story of his or her life. The principles applied to understanding the nodes of the functional biological systems and how imbalances within these nodes challenge system-wide homeostasis, tip the scale, and lead to illness, apply here. A major contributing factor is not our genes, but our environment, including lifestyle, which leads to the imbalances within each of the individual nodes. For example, an article published in the *Journal of the American Medical Association* suggests that 45.4% of cardiometabolic deaths in the United States in 2012 were due to dietary factors alone, such as excess sodium intake, insufficient intake of nuts and seeds, high intake of processed meats, and low intake of omega-3 fats[45].

Barbie's migraine story can be re-told using a functional medicine framework. Her family history is notable for migraines, depression, anxiety, hypertension, and heart disease. These antecedent factors are not merely a matter of genetics, however. Genes are passed from generation to generation, and the manner in which genes are expressed under similar environmental conditions can also be passed along. Taking this further, the ability to identify those environmental conditions can be a powerful tool in guiding patients in an alternative direction, away from the factors promoting their illnesses.

Continuing with her timeline, Barbie is the second of three siblings. Her mother was in her mid-twenties when she was born. The pregnancy was uneventful. Her mother took a prenatal vitamin throughout pregnancy, but no medications. Barbie was born full term, in a natural delivery. Her mother tried breastfeeding, but it did not go well, and within a few weeks, Barbie was switched to formula. She had colic. She had recurrent ear infections and strep throat as a child, and was treated with antibiotics on several occasions. She got motion sickness when riding in a car. Her parents were both educated professionals and held their children to high standards. This personality trait was shared by Barbie. She was a good student, and was obsessed with completing her school work and presenting her parents with good grades. They ate the standard American diet, including lots of meat, processed foods for convenience, added salt, dairy, grains, few fruits and vegetables, and not much fiber. She suffered from gastrointestinal symptoms, intermittent diarrhea and constipation, especially around times of family stress or when she had a difficult homework assignment or test. Her pediatrician diagnosed her with Irritable Bowel Syndrome. She had, and still does have, seasonal allergies, and allergies to pet dander, eggs and peanuts. She grew up in an old house, and when the weather was damp she noticed a mold odor in their basement. Barbie's after-school activities included soccer, and there were a few times when she took a ball to the head or collided with another player and "saw stars." She had her first menstrual period at 13 years old, and about a year later experienced her first migraine.

To the patient and her family, there was no clear trigger, except that the headaches first occurred at the beginning of each cycle, and later occurred independent of her menses. She missed school and other activities when she had a particularly bad attack. As an adult, she would lose at least 6 hours (if not the whole day) of productive work. She saw her pediatrician and a specialist for her headaches, and was placed on medication that did help to reduce their frequency for a number of years, but she has never been able to reduce them below four attacks per month. She has some additional medication to treat acute attacks when they come on, but the drug takes at least two hours to work, and is not always effective. Barbie graduated from college and went into law school. She is now an attorney in a large law firm, where the work is demanding. She is married and has one child, but she and her husband had a hard time conceiving after their first child was born. Barbie's periods became irregular, and she had a spontaneous miscarriage. Between work and family life, she finds little time for exercise and she "feels lucky" if she can get seven hours of sleep per night.

The timeline of Barbie's life brings into focus a number of factors that play important roles in the onset and perpetuation of her migraines. In the language of functional medicine, these are called antecedents, triggers, and mediators. Antecedents are factors, genetic or acquired, that predispose to illness. Triggers are factors that tip the homeostatic balance of health during a person's lifetime. They can be events in one's life, or they can be reflected by the signs or symptoms of illness. Mediators are like the triggers, but they are the factors that go on after the onset of illness that tend to maintain the affected individual on his or her trajectory. If we look at Barbie from this perspective, her antecedents include the family history of migraines, depression, and anxiety. Triggers consist of bottle feeding, colic, ear and throat infections, antibiotic exposure, pressure to achieve, the history of irritable bowel syndrome, diet, allergies, mold exposure, concussion, and hormonal fluctuations associated with menstruation. Mediators include diet, high stress job, hormone imbalance leading to spontaneous miscarriage and irregular menstrual periods, current diet, lack of exercise, and variable sleep quality. Based on an understanding of the functional biological systems described in the previous chapter, it is possible to imagine imbalances in Assimilation, Defense & Repair, Energy, Communication, and Structural Integrity, for example. Problems might include imbalances in the gut microbial community, increased gut and blood-brain barrier permeability, a pro-inflammatory state, poor antioxidant capacity and impaired mitochondrial function. Now, the challenge is to help Barbie get better, to regain her brain health and vitality.

As a physician, the technique of gathering and organizing the timeline utilizes the strengths of motivational interviewing. The history is patient-centered, rather than disease-centered. The approach allows the interviewer to act as a facilitator in the process. As Barbie tells her own story, she gains insight, and those insights are further reinforced with the interviewer summarizing and retelling of the story back to her in the end, highlighting the most important points. The goal is to move her to a point of understanding, then one of action.

If we return to the conventional experience of a visit to the doctor, the most that a patient like Barbie might be asked to do is to try one or two medications to improve her migraines. While there are serious considerations regarding cost, inconvenience, and the potential for side effects that need to be taken into account when accepting a drug as treatment, for the most part, Barbie's role is passive in this scenario. All she needs to do is open her mouth, pop in a pill, swallow it, and wait for the drug to improve her situation, if it does so at all.

With the functional medicine approach, she may be nurtured through a number of pivotal changes in her life. A deeper examination of factors surrounding sleep, nutrition, exercise, and stress resilience will need to take place, for her to change the trajectory of her illness. Furthermore, a knowledge of the nodes that make up the clinical imbalances will allow for a deeper dive, greater insight, and targeted management where needed. Outcomes can be tracked using a variety of instruments, such as headache or symptoms burden questionnaires, along with laboratory imbalances that need to be corrected.

CHAPTER 7

Getting Around the Parts of the Brain

How Structure Relates to Function, When it Comes to Preventing Memory Loss

"No memory is ever alone; it's at the end of a trail of memories, a dozen trails that each have their own associations."

—Louis L'Amour, writer

I first met Doug when he was referred to my office by his primary care physician, who was concerned about progressive memory loss. At the time of our initial visit, he was 67 years old, and self-employed. He performed home appraisals. Over the past two years, he had become increasingly aware of difficulty in functioning, both personally and professionally. He had gotten confused while performing his job, and had to start all over again. "I could not remember what I was doing," he said. He struggled with the math when calculating his estimates. Navigating his way around large homes became increasingly tedious. He would forget specific appraisal contracts he had discussed, and even the names of professional colleagues he had known for years. There was occasional word-finding difficulty. He knew what he wanted to say, but would have trouble expressing the right words, interrupt his speech, or sometimes say the wrong word altogether. After the day at work, he would return home, and would become agitated easily with minor nuisances around the house. This was a change in his personality. He seemed depressed, and sleep was restless. Doug's doctor sent him for an MRI of the brain, which showed moderate atrophy, meaning loss of brain volume, in the area known as the hippocampus.

In order to put together all the pieces of Doug's brain-protecting strategy, it is necessary to have a primer on brain anatomy, and identify the different regions involved with neurological conditions. We can begin with the two cerebral hemispheres — right and left — that make up a large part of the human brain. Each hemisphere is divided into four lobes. The frontal lobe contains nerve cells involved with voluntary movement of the different parts of the body, the production of language, mood, personality, and higher order thinking such as planning, attention, decision-making, and motivation. The part of the frontal lobe involved with movement is called the Primary Motor Cortex. This area contains nerve cells called upper motor neurons, and the combined degeneration of these neurons with the motor neurons in the peripheral nerves outside of the spinal cord (called lower motor neurons) is what causes Amyotrophic Lateral Sclerosis (ALS), or Lou Gehrig's disease. Damage to these upper motor neurons causes spasticity, a stiffness or tightness of muscles that can be obvious to the point of rigidity, or subtle, as when it is only noticeable if the limb is moved. Spasticity is not exclusive to ALS. Anything that disrupts these upper motor neurons can cause spasticity. In other words, to gain greater insight into what is going on with the brain, it is just as important to understand *where* the damage is occurring as *what* has caused that damage. This concept is called "localization," and it is one of the key distinguishing features of neurology. Neurologists use their knowledge of anatomy to "localize" the area of abnormality before they consider the list of possible causes.

Behind the frontal lobes are the parietal lobes, which receive sensory information from the body. This is the area of the primary sensory cortex for pressure, touch, temperature, and pain. But the parietal lobes also integrate sensory information to give it greater meaning, such as "I feel sharp pain at the elbow of what I recognize as my left arm." A fascinating syndrome affecting individuals with damage to the right parietal lobe is known as spatial neglect. In this situation, they may fail to recognize objects placed in the left side of their vision, even when they can see. In some cases, they may not even recognize that a left arm or hand, when presented to the right visual field, belongs to them. It is as if the entire left side of their world does not exist. Further back, beyond the parietal lobes, are the occipital lobes, which serve as the visual cortex, interpreting information received from the eyes. Finally, the temporal lobes, each located on the sides of the hemispheres, process information for hearing and, generally on the left, the recognition of language. The side of the brain on which language is processed and expressed is called the dominant hemisphere.

Other important parts of the brain include the cerebellar hemispheres, at the back of the brain, which help coordinate muscle movements and posture. The brainstem connects the spinal cord to the cerebral hemispheres and cerebellum. It is dense with nerve fibers from the face, head, and body, and divided into three parts: the medulla, pons, and midbrain. The brainstem also has a region known as the reticular activating system, responsible for regulating the level of consciousness. Just above the brainstem is the thalamus, a switching station or relay for descending nerve impulses from the hemispheres and impulses from sensors and nerves in the body that need to be directed to higher areas in the brain.

Deep within the cerebral hemispheres are several other critical brain regions. The basal ganglia is the term for a group of structures collectively involved with control of voluntary movement, especially learned movement and movements that are habitual or unconscious. I always think of the paper rolls that holds the information about which keys to play, and for how long, on an old player piano. The motor cortex of the cerebral hemispheres sends the command to activate a muscle, but the basal ganglia structures express that movement as something meaningful, while the cerebellum helps to make sure that the movement is smooth, coordinated, and graceful. The structures that make up the basal ganglia have names like the caudate nucleus, putamen, globus pallidus, substantia nigra, and subthalamic nucleus.

The basal ganglia is affected in Parkinson's disease, when dopamine-producing cells of the substantia nigra die off through apoptosis. Inflammation and oxidative stress, and the factors that drive these two processes, hold the key to understanding why these normal cellular operations occurs to the point of detriment. Hopefully, what you have learned so far in this book has given you insight into Parkinson's disease from a root cause perspective. A number of other neurological disorders localize to the basal ganglia, including Tourette's syndrome and Huntington's disease.

Several glandular structures are located within the brain. The pineal gland produces melatonin, synthesized from the neurotransmitter serotonin. Among this hormone's roles is regulation of the sleep-wake cycle by helping to set the body's internal clock.

The pituitary gland sits inside a boney cave on the underside of the brain. It forms a feedback loop with other glands located in the body, including the thyroid gland, ovaries and testes, and the adrenal glands, by increasing its release of gland-stimulating hormones when the brain detects levels are low, and decreasing the release of gland-stimulating hormones when levels are high. The hypothalamus, a brain region adjacent to the pituitary gland, works in coordination with the pituitary to act as a link between the nervous system and the glands of the body, and provide a higher degree of control over the release of hormones. It serves a wide range of functions. The hypothalamus regulates the release of pituitary hormones that signal the ovaries and testes to produce estrogen and testosterone. It signals the thyroid to secrete its hormone. It regulates body temperature, water balance, blood pressure, heart rate, pupil size, perspiration, hunger, feeding and satiety. The hypothalamus is involved in learning, memory, sleep and arousal. It releases the hormone oxytocin, which has a diversity of functions, including its role in human bonding, dilation of the cervix during childbirth, and the milk letdown reflex when breastfeeding.

As a regulatory center, the hypothalamus can direct lower levels of cortisol hormone to be released from the adrenal glands after a period of sustained cortisol elevation. This is an adaptive response, a pattern of homeostasis that protects us, sometimes to the detriment of how we might feel. This phenomenon is common in pain conditions like fibromyalgia and chronic fatigue.

Abnormal activity from the hypothalamus has also been associated with the sleep disorder narcolepsy with cataplexy. This condition is thought to have an autoimmune basis, and is characterized by persistent sleepiness, sudden loss of muscle tone triggered by strong emotion, episodes of paralysis upon awakening, and vivid hallucinations while falling asleep or waking up.

As our journey circles back toward our patient Doug, it is necessary to visit one more group of structures in the middle of the brain collectively known as the limbic system. The limbic system includes the thalamus, hypothalamus, cingulate gyrus, amygdala, hippocampus, and fornix (which connects the hippocampus to the hypothalamus). Together, these structures play a role in our most primal instincts involving emotions, like fear, anxiety, depression, aggression, motivation, pleasure, reward and impulse behavior, sexual behavior, navigation, learning, and memory. Fundamentally, the limbic system is connected to individual and species survival, instinctive self-preservation, self-propagating, and protection behaviors. With its primal roots, the limbic system is also tied to our sense of smell, and the olfactory bulbs — our smell detecting cranial nerves — not surprisingly, are considered part of the limbic system.

The hippocampus, which showed moderate atrophy in Doug's brain, is a structure located on the medial aspect of each of the temporal lobes. It is said to resemble a seahorse. The hippocampus is particularly known for its central role in Alzheimer's disease, first described by the German physician Dr. Aloysius Alzheimer in 1901. The patient, a woman named Auguste Deter, no longer able to receive care from her husband, was committed to the Frankfurt City Hospital for the Mentally Ill and Epileptics. She presented with severe cognitive decline, hallucinations, language difficulty, and behavioral changes. After she died in 1906, Dr. Alzheimer, whose focus bridged psychiatry and neuropathology, examined Frau Deter's brain under the microscope and noted two changes, *neurofibrillary tangles* and *amyloid plaques*. These neurofibrillary tangles are actually the remnants of a transport system within nerve cells that, under normal conditions, moves nutrients and other essential supplies along the length of the cell, from the cell body down the axon. These transport systems are known as microtubules, and a protein called tau plays a role in stabilizing the microtubule structure. In the context of Alzheimer's disease, the tau protein becomes phosphorylated, which means a phosphate group is added onto the protein, and the result disrupts the microtubule organization, causing clumps to form (the neurofibrillary tangle). This renders the cell unable to function, and ultimately leads to its demise.

The plaques are the other half of the Alzheimer's story. These plaques are composed of a specific protein known as amyloid beta-42, where the "42" refers to the number of amino acids that make up its length. The configuration of this amyloid is formed from a parent protein ubiquitous throughout the body, found tethered to the surface membrane of cells, in what are termed "lipid rafts." In the brain, this Amyloid Precursor Protein (APP) is found on neurons, where its role in making and grooming the connection between nerve cells positions it as a major player in the process of neuroplasticity (a broad term that describes the ability of the brain to change or adapt, and includes the capacity for learning and memory). The cell, able to detect signals within its environment, can activate enzymes, based on those signals, which cut or process this Amyloid Precursor Protein in different ways. The result of this processing of APP can be amyloid beta-42 and other proteins which have been shown to limit the growth of nerve cell axons, their ability to make connections with other neurons, and trigger apoptosis. Conversely, if the APP is cut or processed into other proteins, such as sAPPα (α is the Greek letter alpha) the result is proteins which promote survival, nerve branch growth, and improve memory function. Like other aspects of biological function, this is a matter of homeostasis and the factors that tip this balance in one direction or another (allostasis), namely, those which drive inflammation and oxidative stress.

Complicating this further is a gene for a class of proteins whose job it is to transport cholesterol and phospholipids to nerve cells. This gene, known as ApoE, codes for apolipoprotein epsilon. Within the population, there are three known forms of these genes, known as ApoE2, ApoE3, and ApoE4. In 1993, a Duke University neuroscientist, Dr. Alan Roses, reported that carriers of the ApoE4 variant have a significantly increased risk of Alzheimer's disease later in life (after age 65), and the risk goes up depending on whether a person has one or two copies of this gene[46]. Each of us gets one copy from our mother and one copy from our father. ApoE4 is found in about 20-30 percent of the population in the United States, for example, and those who have one copy have approximately twice the risk of developing the disease, whereas those with two copies have up to 12 times the risk of Alzheimer's disease. While carriers of the ApoE3 subtype can still get Alzheimer's disease, their risk is not considered above the population norm. ApoE2 appears to confer a degree of protection against the development of the disease (unless paired with ApoE4). ApoE4 strongly influences the production of amyloid beta-42 in the brain. What appears to be promoting these effects on the nerve cell? The answer is those drivers of neuroinflammation: signals from the gut, infections, toxins, excess oxidative stress, nutrient depletion, hormone imbalances, head trauma, emotional or psychological stress (through the limbic system). While ApoE4 status is not the sole determinant of Alzheimer's disease, it does increase the risk and the need to be especially vigilant about addressing imbalances within the functional biological systems that affect the health of the brain.

PART 2
THE STRATEGIES

CHAPTER 8

Brain Tune Up! In the Office

How a Functional Medicine Practice Can Work for You

"A self that is only differentiated — not integrated — may attain great individual accomplishments, but risks being mired in self-centered egotism. By the same token, a person whose self is based exclusively on integration will be well-connected and secure, but lack autonomous individuality. Only when a person invests equal amounts of psychic energy in these two processes and avoids both selfishness and conformity is the self likely to reflect complexity."

—Mihaly Csikszentmihalyi, psychologist and author

What you are about to learn are the principles I teach my patients in my office-based functional medicine program, *Brain Tune Up!* For the past 5 years, through a combination of education, trial and error, I have refined my approach to brain health and created a successful program that helps multitudes of people prevent or reverse memory loss, and protect their aging brains. My team and I have witnessed the turnabout of illnesses that are supposed to be chronic and progressive, and in some cases fatal. This includes Alzheimer's disease, Parkinson's disease, Amyotrophic Lateral Sclerosis, Multiple Sclerosis, migraines, and Fibromyalgia. The framework of *Brain Tune Up!* was shared with you in **Part 1** of this book. Now you are going to learn how to apply the principles of *Brain Tune Up!* into a practical system that you can use for the rest of your life.

There are no compromises. I will show you that the use of lifestyle-based strategies is the most potent medicine we have, to combat the downward spiral of chronic disease. Our current medical culture wants us to "swallow the pill," literally and figuratively, that chronic disease of the brain is a consequence of the aging process, part of "normal aging," and that it is necessary to accept these conditions as we get older. Sleep, movement and exercise; nutrition; mental, emotional, and spiritual resilience; and nurturing relationships are at the foundation of brain health. While more advanced strategies are possible, the foundation of lifestyle is an absolute requirement for success. The floors, walls, and roof of a home cannot be constructed until the foundation is built, and so it is with a successful strategy to prevent memory loss and protect the aging brain. I am often asked by patients who visit my office, interested in doing something good for themselves but unfamiliar with functional medicine, whether I can "treat them naturally." They mean that I should suggest a management strategy for their condition in which supplements — vitamins and herbs — are used, in lieu of medication. I will never forget one family that brought their father to see me when he had advanced Alzheimer's disease. They had large shopping bags full of supplement bottles. I took them out of the bags, lined them side-by-side on my examination table, and the length of the row of bottles exceeded the six foot length of the table. Aside from the enormous cost of these supplements, the unfortunate result of all this effort was that the patient had not gained anything meaningful as a result of using them. In fact, he likely lost precious time because he put his faith in these pills while he waited for them to make his brain better; instead, he continued to deteriorate and unfortunately reached a point where little could be done to guide him back to a state of resilient health.

This is not intended to discredit supplements. I recommend high quality supplements in my office on a regular basis. They have value when used in a targeted manner when deficiencies or other imbalances are identified, or when a specific therapeutic effect is the goal. Furthermore, in Chapter 13, I will tell you which ones I think may have value in a self-directed plan like *The Healthy Brain Toolbox*, and why.

In my *Brain Tune Up!* office program, once my patients have embraced the idea of change through functional medicine, they start the process by completing a lengthy questionnaire on the computer, and scheduling an appointment to go over their <u>functional medicine timeline</u>. This is the story of the patient's life, from pre-birth to birth, childhood through adulthood. Using this technique to elicit the information populates their timeline, reflects back the most critical points, and when the story is retold, it empowers them to make changes using lifestyle, targeted supplementation, and holistic medicine strategies.

An understanding of the areas of clinical imbalance is also facilitated by the neurological and nutritional physical examination. I perform the neurological examination, and my dietician performs a nutritional physical examination with particular attention to hair, skin, mouth, eyes, and nails for clues about possible nutritional deficiencies or imbalances. We measure height, weight, body mass index, core temperature, blood pressure, pulse, and respirations. The same day, the patient undergoes an extensive battery of blood tests, which will be reviewed with them when the results are available a few weeks later.

The blood tests can be grouped into categories which highlight their relevance to different areas of clinical imbalance, as represented by the functional biological systems: Nutrients and Digestive Markers (Assimilation), Inflammatory and Infectious Markers (Defense & Repair), Heavy Metals and Liver Enzymes (Biotransformation & Elimination), Antioxidants (Energy), Hormones (Communication). Blood tests for Structural Integrity and Transport are not performed in my clinic. But patients do have a physical examination for structural imbalance and, if necessary, magnetic resonance (MRA), computed tomographic angiography (CTA), or ultrasound, can be ordered to evaluate blood vessel integrity.

Sometimes, too, patients undergo additional diagnostic testing in the beginning of the program because they have not been thoroughly evaluated for the conditions they believe they have. This may be because they have diagnosed themselves, or they have been given a diagnosis by another practitioner who has not performed a thorough evaluation. For example, I have seen patients self-referred for Alzheimer's disease who, despite having memory difficulty, did not have evidence of Alzheimer's disease. These patients may undergo spinal fluid testing for amyloid beta-42, tau, and phosphorylated tau protein, volumetric brain imaging using magnetic resonance imaging (MRI) technology augmented with additional software called NeuroQuant®, Brain Positron Emission Tomography (PET), and genetic testing.

There are other disease mimics. Parkinsonism includes other neurodegenerative disorders, can be confused for essential tremor, and medication-induced parkinsonism. Multiple sclerosis is a frequent go-to diagnosis when a young person presents with a spectrum of unusual or difficult to measure symptoms, and their MRI of the brain shows nonspecific changes. There are diseases that can present with similar distinguishing features, such as Lyme disease, B12 deficiency, and CADASIL[47]. While fibromyalgia, chronic fatigue, headaches, and depression are symptoms-based diagnoses, it is still helpful to make sure that something has not been missed, such as Obstructive Sleep Apnea (a disorder in which the upper airway closes off during sleep and results in a significant drop in blood oxygen) or a hormone imbalance disorder.

Even though functional medicine is about helping my patients identify and address the root causes of their conditions, I think it is helpful and necessary to make sure to know where we are starting. I call the downstream diagnosis the "anchoring point."

Lastly, because functional medicine is also about having the outcomes you want, tracking tools are routinely used to measure a baseline and repeat over time to document progress. Two commonly used tracking tools are the <u>Medical Symptoms Questionnaire</u> (MSQ) and the <u>Montreal Cognitive Assessment</u> (MoCA). The version of the MSQ used in my clinic is from The Institute for Functional Medicine. Here, the link to the MSQ is credited to Dr. Mark Hyman, physician and author, pioneer in functional medicine, and former Chairman of the Board of Directors at IFM.

The final point to keep in mind is the notion that these lifestyle factors, like the functional biological systems, are connected to and influence one another. Food, for example, is a critical part of this brain health plan, but a successful approach to preventing memory loss and protecting your aging brain involves more than food. If my patients focus on food only, and do not address the important roles that sleep, movement and exercise, emotional and psychological stress resilience, and relationships play in this lifestyle-based functional medicine approach, they will not get better. The "art" of functional medicine for the brain is how the individual pieces of the puzzle are integrated and nurtured along in a stepwise, achievable fashion, in a realistic manner that can be accomplished based on the uniqueness of each individual who makes this approach their focus.

CHAPTER 9

Sleep Is More Than A Time Of Rest

Get Your Zzzs to Protect Your Brain!

"Sleep is that golden chain that ties health and our bodies together."

—Thomas Dekker, actor and musician

When Shakespeare's Hamlet uttered the famous line, "to sleep, perchance to dream," he was actually talking about death and the possibility that he might be locked in a perpetual and disturbing dream state, in the afterlife. Nevertheless, the line is a segue to recognize the importance of sleep to the balance and optimization of the functional biological systems, and to make sure every individualized program includes a focus on sleep.

Sleep is much more than a period of rest, the need to close our eyes, and the desire to feel refreshed upon awakening. It is a period of remarkable biological activity. Sleep plays a critical role in digestion and absorption of nutrients, gut microbial balance, the clearing of toxins through the glymphatic system, and immune function. Shift workers, whose job it is to work overnight, disrupt normal sleep function, and may have greater risk of infection and autoimmune disorders[48]. In a mouse experiment on sleep apnea, the periods of low blood oxygen caused by the pauses in breathing was found to alter the balance of gut bacteria. The mice had a more abundant bacterium known as *Firmicutes*, and fewer bacteria known as *Bacteroidetes*[49]. In humans, evidence suggests that the gut bacteria composition is different in lean individuals, compared to obese individuals who have a higher *Firmicutes* to *Bacteroidetes* ratio, and a similar effect can be mimicked in lean individuals subjected to sleep deprivation[50]. While being overweight is associated with the risk of sleep apnea in the first place, sleep apnea may also promote a balance of bacteria that causes weight gain or makes it harder to lose weight. Sleep protects brain cells, such as those of the hippocampus, by ensuring that a sufficient supply of antioxidants is available to protect the mitochondria from excess oxidative stress. Growth hormone and testosterone, essential to repair and restoration of brain tissue, are secreted during sleep. Those affected by poor quality sleep may experience a decrease in these hormones and an increase in the stress hormone cortisol. This increase in cortisol, in turn, disrupts sleep, raises glucose and insulin levels, and contributes to the risk of obesity, insulin resistance, and diabetes.

Perhaps most important to this book's message of preventing memory loss, sleep is a time the brain uses to organize and store memory. The process of sleep influences what information gets saved as long-term memory. The stage of sleep known as REM or Rapid Eye Movement sleep benefits memory related to how we do things ("procedural memory") while non-REM sleep benefits memory related to facts and events ("declarative memory"). Tasks learned during one day are better performed the next day after a good night of sleep, and significantly better performed than after a night of no sleep at all. REM sleep may facilitate creativity, reasoning, and higher-level insights (those "Ah-ha!" moments). Sleep affects mood. We all know that a good night of sleep gives us better control over our emotions. We just feel good after a solid night of sleep!

Human beings, like other animals, have built-in biological clocks called "circadian clocks" that help determine our timing of sleep. The main circadian clock that governs the sleep-wake cycle is located in the hypothalamus. Although it runs independently, it is adjusted by external cues, so that its timing remains accurate. The most important factor that helps to set this clock is daylight. This is why we are actually biologically designed to go to sleep within a couple of hours of sunset. The clock, in turn, regulates not only sleep, but eating patterns, alertness, core body temperature, brain wave activity, hormone production, regulation of glucose and insulin levels, urine production, and other activities. The circadian system sends out an alerting pulse throughout the day. As the alerting pulses start to weaken, the drive to sleep predominates. The pineal gland releases melatonin, the "sleep gate" opens, and the urge to sleep increases dramatically. Besides melatonin, release of the hormone cortisol is controlled by the circadian clock.

Counterbalancing the body's built in sleep-wake clock is a separate process that drives the pressure to sleep as a function of the amount of time elapsed since the last adequate sleep episode. This is called sleep-wake homeostasis, and it follows the principle that we tend to get sleepier as the day goes on. Conversely, the longer we have been asleep, the more the pressure to sleep dissipates, and the more likely we are to awaken. Governing this drive to sleep is a chemical called adenosine, located in an area of the frontal lobes known as the basal forebrain. Adenosine was discussed earlier in the review of mitochondria and energy production in the form of adenosine triphosphate or ATP. It turns out that the adenosine that promotes the urge to sleep is created over the course of the day as a result of our using up our natural energy stores of ATP. This makes sense! Commonly used stimulants, like caffeine in coffee and tea, and theophylline in tea and chocolate, work as adenosine blockers. This is how drinking a cup of your favorite java helps you stay awake.

A number of neurotransmitters are involved in wakefulness and sleep. Among these, histamine is sometimes referred to as the "master" wakefulness-promoting neurotransmitter. When histamine is blocked, we feel sleepy. This is why over-the-counter antihistamines are sold as sleep aids (those "PM"-brand medications). While nearly every neurotransmitter found in the brain has a role in sleep or wakefulness, two others are worth mentioning. Gamma Aminobutyric Acid, or GABA, the main inhibitory neurotransmitter in the brain, plays an essential role in promoting the onset of sleep by inhibiting the firing of cells involved in wakefulness, such as histamine-producing cells. Medications known as benzodiazepines (such as diazepam and alprazolam) and other prescription sleeping pills work through GABA. Another important chemical in the sleep-wake cycle is orexin, a neurotransmitter that regulates arousal, wakefulness, and appetite. It is produced by specialized nerve cells in the hypothalamus, although the long axons of these nerves extend throughout the entire brain and spinal cord. Activation of orexin triggers wakefulness, while low levels promote sleep. Orexin deficiency results in sleep disorders like narcolepsy, which appear to have an autoimmune basis — in other words, when orexin-producing cells are destroyed by the immune system.

How can these principles be used to improve sleep and promote a healthy brain? First and foremost, it is important to get enough sleep, generally 7-8 hours per night. Try to keep a regular sleep schedule and go to sleep within 2-3 hours of sunset. Dim the lights in your home after the sun has gone down by turning off unnecessary fixtures. Blue light is composed of the visible wavelengths we call daylight, and daylight suppresses melatonin release. Consider using blue light filter lenses, so-called "blue blocker" glasses, or amber bulbs in your home in order to filter the wavelength of light associated with daylight, and therefore wakefulness. Some electronic equipment, such as cell phones, can change screen color at night to emit less blue wavelength. Similarly, you can install programs like f.lux to alter the light of your computer screen at night.

Here are some other strategies to induce sleepiness. Reduce noise and create an atmosphere of calm. If necessary, a low dose of melatonin, 0.5 to 3 mg for adults, may be used to trigger a sense of sleepiness. Consider a warm bath with Epsom salt. The cooling of your body after the warm bath mimics the drop in body temperature that accompanies the onset of sleep. The magnesium in Epsom salt helps regulate brain signals that lead to the secretion of cortisol and the other stress hormone, epinephrine, by the adrenal glands. While GABA itself is poorly absorbed from the gut, teas with valerian root and chamomile contain active compounds that stimulate GABA receptors, and can make you sleepy. Keep your bedroom cool, and do not use too many blankets. When we fall asleep, our bodies naturally cool, so try to sleep in a cooler room to maintain a lower body temperature.

Avoid alcohol at night. You may fall asleep more quickly, but it alters the structure of sleep and may cause you to wake up in the early morning hours. It can also worsen sleep apnea.

If there is a suspicion of sleep apnea, be sure to get checked by a sleep specialist and have a sleep test called a polysomnogram. Sleep apnea is a serious health problem, and can contribute to the risk of heart attack, stroke, Alzheimer's disease, and premature death. Treat it right away!

Sleep apnea is not the only cause of Excessive Daytime Sleepiness (EDS). EDS can be caused by the disease narcolepsy. Take the Epworth Sleepiness Scale Test to determine your level of sleepiness. Any score above 10 is consistent with EDS where 11-2 is considered mild, 13-15 moderate, and 16-20 severe. Severe EDS, in particular, is associated with an increased risk of motor vehicle crashes.

As a condition that affects 30% of adults, insomnia (difficulty either falling asleep or maintaining sleep) can occur for many reasons. It can be due to a noisy environment, poor habits, such as consuming stimulants (like coffee) too late in the day, a variety of physical illnesses, such as diabetes, heart disease, acid reflux, thyroid disorders, lung disease, or those that cause chronic pain. Some medications can contribute to insomnia. The list includes certain antidepressants, medications for Parkinson's disease, blood pressure medications, and prednisone. Please check with your doctor if you think your medication is causing you insomnia. Psychological factors, including stressful circumstances, anxiety, depression, or a tendency to ruminate contribute to insomnia, as well. A powerful tool called Cognitive Behavioral Therapy (CBT) is highly effective for insomnia. CBT involves helping people to change the way they think or behave as a way to manage their circumstances. Two excellent resources for CBT include this <u>search engine</u> for therapists trained in the technique, and <u>SHUTi,</u> an online self-directed subscription-based program. Exercise, change in dietary habits, and relaxation techniques are also important when it comes to addressing insomnia, and these will be covered in the chapters to come.

CHAPTER 10

Movement and Exercise

How Physical Activity Prevents Memory Loss and Protects Your Brain

Guest Author: Amy Gordin, PT

"Human bodies are designed for regular physical activity. The sedentary nature of much of modern life probably plays a significant role in the epidemic incidence of depression today. Many studies show that depressed patients who stick to a regimen of aerobic exercise improve as much as those treated with medication."

—Andrew Weil, MD, holistic physician and author

T he *Brain Tune Up!* program at Sharlin Health and Neurology in Ozark, Missouri employs a team-based approach. The next three chapters, including this chapter on exercise, are written by guest authors who are members of my team. These lifestyle medicine professionals each put their unique signatures on the *Brain Tune Up!* experience for those who come from all over the world to visit us. I am pleased to share their wisdom with you in this book.

Amy Gordin, PT is a graduate of the University of Missouri. She is a license physical therapist who has completed additional training with the American Council on Exercise, and in TRX, Crossfit Level 1, Crossfit Mobility, and Crossfit Kids. Amy is the founder of Sessions, a functional movement and exercise facility in Nixa, Missouri. She brings tremendous enthusiasm to her work, and has made many "converts" to the exercise lifestyle through her infectious energy and joy in what she does. Before we hear from Amy, I am going to provide some background.

It may be no coincidence that the most recent recommendations from the American Academy of Neurology, entitled *Practice Guideline Update: Mild Cognitive Impairment*, recommends exercise training as the #1 lifestyle strategy to improve memory loss and protect the aging brain[51]. In 2012, Lindsay Nagamatsu and her colleagues published an article in *JAMA Internal Medicine* (formerly *Archives of Internal Medicine*), entitled "Resistance Training Promotes Cognitive and Functional Brain Plasticity in Seniors with Probable Mild Cognitive Impairment[52]." The report was a randomized trial designed to provide evidence that both resistance training and cardiovascular exercises could improve cognitive functioning in adults at risk for developing Alzheimer's disease. They wanted to know whether both types of exercise could improve memory performance, everyday problem-solving, and overall physical function. The average age of study participants was 75. These researchers demonstrated that twice weekly resistance training showed improvement across multiple outcome measures. In addition, the cardiovascular training improved physical functions such as balance, mobility, and cardiovascular capacity. In a separate paper published one year later in *PLOS ONE*, Takao Suzuki and colleagues reported on a randomized control trial of multi-component exercise in older adults with mild cognitive impairment. They found that exercise improved logical memory and helped to maintain cognitive function, while reducing whole brain atrophy[53]. There were twice-weekly exercise classes. Each 90 minute class began with a 10 minute warm up period and stretching exercise, followed by 20 minutes of muscle strength, then cardiovascular exercises (stair stepping, endurance walking or walking), postural balance training such as walking on balance boards, and dual task training — walking while inventing their own poems. Some of the classes included outdoor walking. Participants had independent home training, which involved both strength exercises and walking.

Not surprisingly, exercise has a positive effect on every one of the functional biological systems discussed in **Part 1** of this book. Exercise alters the gut microbiome, encouraging both diversity and development of beneficial bacteria. Exercise for as little as 20 minutes can boost your immune system. (But be careful, because overdoing it can actually damage immune function.) Exercise protects mitochondria by increasing the capacity for mitochondria to manage those reactive oxygen species we discussed in the section on oxidative stress, while at the same time, it triggers the formation of new mitochondria. Exercise helps to detoxify the body through sweat, respiration, improved bowel and bladder function, and by reducing body fat burden, where fat is a harbor of fat-soluble toxins. Exercise is a form of stress that can, in turn, modify the body's response to stress. Once again, it is all about proper dosage, but exercise affects multiple hormones, including cortisol, cytokines, endorphins, growth hormone, testosterone, epinephrine, norepinephrine, and others. Exercise strengthens muscles, tendons, ligaments, joints, and bones, and exercise improves blood flow and stimulates the growth of new blood vessels.

Now, please welcome Amy Gordin:

Hopefully, we have your attention, and you are convinced that exercise is a key part of any program aimed at preventing memory loss and protecting the brain. The good news, too, is that when you exercise for the brain, you are improving every system in your body — organ systems like your heart, and the functional biological systems that have been discussed by Dr. Sharlin earlier in this book.

When it comes to exercise, it can be overwhelming to know where to start. The most effective exercise program begins with an assessment. This is vital to unlock the keys to success and allows me to determine the strengths and weaknesses of my clients. By focusing on strengths, in particular, I can meet individuals at their current levels, and build on a foundation of enthusiasm and ability. If a 78 year old client played basketball in high school, this information is used to create an exercise program that begins with the age and ability-appropriate movements reminiscent of that sport. For example, I might have him shuffle between cones while tossing him a basketball. This is a fun way to challenge balance and agility. If a 50 year old woman with memory loss enjoyed dance in her youth, I might use braiding (also called grapevine) in her program to give her confidence when teaching her new exercises. Braiding is a technique reminiscent of dance[54]. When a 17 year old says that she hates to run, it is important to use other options when I introduce exercises to increase her heart rate. Once I gain the trust and confidence of my clients, they begin to see strength and fitness result. Then I introduce those less desirable activities in small doses, and their mental roadblocks fall away.

The significance of the medical history cannot be overstated. Do you have a history of cervical spine fusion? If you do, we might want to talk about a neutral spine. (This is when all three natural curves of the spine are in alignment, which creates a position of strength and stability.) You may need to minimize overhead activities. Instead, postural awareness will be a focus of your exercise prescription. Maybe you have limited yourself because of outdated advice? For example, I had a client with a history of back injury tell me that his physician told him not to lift over 10 pounds. Upon further investigation, I discovered that this restriction was imposed 40 years ago. We were able to get medical clearance for him to go above this limit and build critical strength. Another client I saw recently was told by her physician not to squat. Maybe the physician actually meant not to perform *weighted* squats, but the client was afraid to perform all squats, even air squats, a squat movement that does not involve weights.

One of the most important pieces of the puzzle is the reason the client is in my gym. As a trainer, I need to understand the motivation. Why do they want to start an exercise program? Because my clients use exercise as medicine, there is a variety of reasons they seek my help. It may be that they have a family member who has been diagnosed with diabetes, and their own fear of insulin injections brought them to me. It could be that someone has hit rock bottom emotionally, and seeks relief from anxiety and depression through exercise. It could be a client whose physical decline has made it impossible for him to pursue his passion for flying airplanes, or another who is unable to get on the floor to play with grandchildren. When that grandmother wants to give up during a workout, a quick reminder of her underlying motivation, her grandchildren, is an instant energy boost. Perhaps the reason for following an exercise prescription is that you want to improve your brain health? I suspect that's the case! Whatever the reason, the underlying motivation can be used to facilitate change for the better.

The easiest part of the assessment is the physical abilities testing. In *Brain Tune Up!*, the assessment starts with an evaluation of <u>squat form</u>, <u>maximum plank time</u>, and <u>push-ups</u>. Often times, the medical history will lead to additional tests. For instance, a client that explains she has difficulty getting out of a low chair would perform a <u>30 second chair rise</u> in order to measure her current abilities and ensure future progress. The squat is critical to activities of daily living, and squat errors can lead to a multitude of problems. If a client says she has knee problems, is it common to find excessive anterior translation of the knees during the squat, an improper form in which the knees move over the toes. Or the knees might fall inward, creating a "valgus stress." The client has a huge payoff when he or she fixes this squat issue and sees these knee symptoms improve. Similarly, someone with a history of back pain will benefit from a squat that utilizes a good hip hinge (where the hips move back before the knees bend) and activation of the posterior chain of muscles, consisting of the glutes, hamstrings, calves, and back musculature. The importance of perfecting the squat is critical to adding weight or complexity of exercise. For example, it is impossible to do a good <u>kettlebell swing</u> without good squat form.

<u>Plank time</u> gives good information about core strength and serves as an important tool to measure progress. <u>Push-ups</u> give insight into functional ability, as well. If the spine is unstable during a push up from the ground, it suggests that performing an elevated push up is a better starting point. Although many trainers will modify the push up with knees on the ground, my experience is that it is more difficult to teach clients to stabilize their spines with that technique. Elevating the push up on a large wooden box called a "plyo" found in the gym, or an ottoman at home, can be a safe and effective solution.

Once the basic assessment is done, it is time to prescribe the exercise program itself. The research is clear that intensity is the variable most commonly associated with optimal results. This is the rationale behind High Intensity Interval Training (HIIT). Intensity is responsible for the neuroendocrine response. This refers to the interaction between our hormones and our nervous systems. A HIIT work out of 20 minutes can be far superior to a low intensity walk for an hour. A common application of HIIT is known as Tabata. Dr. Tabata studied Japanese speed skaters in 1996 and discovered this secret — that short bursts of effort can have an exponentially greater benefit for fitness. This involves 20 seconds of high intensity effort, followed by 10 seconds of rest (or lower intensity activity) for a duration of 4 minutes. The neuroendocrine gains persist for up to 48 hours following a HIIT workout. Although this is not the place to start with beginners, it is important to introduce high intensity concepts as soon as possible, and to realize that intensity varies depending on level of fitness. Borrowing from Dr. Tabata, the movements of skating can be adapted to the gym for part of a high intensity workout. Here is how to do <u>skaters</u>.

Our clients are asked to rate their exercise intensity on a scale of 0 to 10. Ten is a maximum effort, in which the client feels like they will pass out or vomit! Don't worry, I encourage my clients to get to the 7 or 8 range. This can be hard to understand if you are new to exercise. Instead, the "talk test" can be used to help explain intensity. If a person can speak in full sentences without difficulty, their intensity is lower than that of someone who can only say a few words without pausing for a breath.

Exercise variability is another key to a successful prescription. The body is quick to adapt to imposed demands. If part of defining fitness is physical adaptability to a variety of activities, then it makes sense to pursue fitness through constant variation. I will bend that rule when working with someone who has significant memory loss. They may have trouble with a lot of variability. For these individuals, I have them do 3 familiar exercises, and add only one new one at a time, to avoid unpleasant confusion. If someone gets frustrated with a new movement, the use of visual cues may be helpful. Performing in front of a mirror may be the answer.

Functional movement is another key component of a good exercise program for the brain. Just as it is impossible to get the multiple benefits of exercise while on the couch, a survey of a typical gym reveals many exercise machines, like bikes and rowers, that ask us to sit and perform an action. The biggest problem is that most of us sit too much, so we don't need to do that in our exercise programs. Another area of concern is that exercise machines typically focus on movement across one joint. This is not how we are designed to move, as human beings.

How do we move in real life situations? Consider a common activity like picking up a laundry basket. We squat down and pick up the basket, then move it to another place. I want movements which cross the midline of the body, alternate between right and left, change directions on command, challenge balance, and use multiple joints! For example, <u>boxing</u> is a great way to incorporate these brain-boosting actions. Asking clients to count their repetitions requires mental focus, and builds that "muscle," too. Depending on the level of difficulty for an individual, it is important that people can get up and down from the floor. It is a predictor of longevity and quality of life, really. Not everyone has to belong to a gym. Some people exercise at home, at the park, or on the trails. Remote training guidance is also possible. I am currently texting workouts to a snowbird couple who will spend the next 3 months in Mexico. Video conferencing software allows for visual guidance and allows me to record the workout routine for playback at a later time.

Community is powerful. I know people can be successful on their own at home with exercise, however I am constantly amazed at the power of the group setting. My group classes that consist of 8 people or fewer still allow for personal attention. In a given group, you would find people of all ages, abilities, and personal physical challenges — individuals with shoulder injuries working out next to people with cognitive impairment. On a daily basis, I see the encouragement that fellow classmates give when they recognize each other's progress. Another way to take advantage of the group setting is to have a workout partner. A good workout can be adapted to challenge the caregiver, as well as someone with cognitive impairment.

When starting with a new client, it is important to expand his or her toolbox. It is common that when people come to me, walking is their only method of exercise. In this case, it is vital to help them increase their knowledge and skill level with a variety of resistance and cardiovascular exercises, and progress to a level of difficulty that truly improves or increases function. To do so, it means I have to meet my clients at their current ability levels, advance difficulty, and increase variability as they show improvement. This may be as simple as adding weight to an exercise or gradually lowering the elevated push up. It may be asking the client to perform a specific circuit faster than they completed it last month. Acquiring new skills often feels like learning a new language.

After several weeks, each client has a long list of exercises that they have mastered and then can use in a variety of circuits. When it comes to designing a circuit, one theory is to start with big muscle groups and progress to smaller muscle groups. squats for the legs, rows for the back, push-ups for the chest and a form of plank for the core. Another option would be retro-lunge for the legs, single-leg row for the back, single-leg press for the upper extremity and bosu Spiderman for the core. It is important to focus on the specific needs of the individual client. If a client spends all day at a computer, his exercise program will need to include shoulder retraction. If there is a history of falls, balance will be emphasized. Additionally, there needs to be feedback about muscle and joint soreness, as another method to determine if exercise can be advanced. Joint pain is a clear indicator of poor form, or of too much, too soon. A bit of muscle soreness is acceptable, and we will continue to advance our programming. But if a client has difficulty getting out of a chair because of muscle soreness, we scale back and add rest days. A client who complains of shoulder soreness can still be advanced with lower extremity exercises, while scaling back or eliminating shoulder-intensive movements. The objective is to provide the optimal exercise stimulus by varying the number of repetitions, surface height, adding weight, or changing the base of support, such as using one leg, versus both legs. Virtually everyone benefits from better strength. On a daily basis, I am reminded of the confidence boost that comes with seeing improvement. This is one of my favorite benefits of exercise, and it is seen with individuals from 8 to 80 years old. Check out the following examples of short, high intensity circuit exercises you can use in your Healthy Brain Toolbox, Circuit 1 and Circuit 2.

CHAPTER 11

Nutrition to Tune Up Your Brain

How Food Provides the Building Blocks to Brain Health

Guest Author: Angela Jenkins, RD, LD

"One cannot think well, love well, sleep well, if one has not dined well."

—Virginia Woolf, writer

Angela Jenkins is a Registered and Licensed Dietitian who has been in practice since 1991. She is the author of the forthcoming *Brain Tune Up! Food and Recipe Guide* for participants in our office-based functional medicine program. Angela's diverse experience includes pediatrics, sports nutrition, and inpatient clinical nutrition in a variety of settings. In 2009, her perspective on food was transformed by a heightened awareness of how food is raised and grown, the influence this has on our health, and the significance that food policy has on our food supply. This was just the first step on a journey that led her outside of a typical dietitian's role. In 2012, she facilitated startup of the Ozarks Regional Food Policy Council in Southwest Missouri. She drew from her experiences in the community, returned to the hospital and clinic setting, and helped her patients improve their health in ways not previously possible. Angela lives on 10 acres in Ozark, Missouri, just a few miles from our clinic, where she is in the process of developing her property into a biodynamic farm. She enjoys staying active. When Angela is not running the Ozark Mountain trails with her dog, Remo, she can be found teaching people how easy it is to produce their own food and prepare it in the comfort of their homes. Her passion can be summed up in a quote from Larry Olmsted, author of *Real Food, Fake Food*: "Like a stone tossed in a pond, deciding what to eat has a ripple effect that goes far beyond the calories needed to carry us from breakfast to lunch to dinner. When you choose to eat real food, your immediate benefit is that it tastes good. In many cases it is also more sustainable, healthier for the environment, and supports people whose work, methods, and entire communities, make the world a better place."

Now, please welcome Angela Jenkins:

What's the big deal with food? According to the United States Department of Agriculture Economic Research Service, consumption of food prepared away from home plays a large role in the American diet. In 2014, this represented 50.1 percent of all household spending on food. Because Americans eat nearly as much food outside the home as inside the home, this creates a setup in our food culture or food environment that leaves half of the decisions about what goes into our bodies to someone else. While we do make the decision about what to choose off of the menu, choices about the ingredients, how they are cooked, and how the food was raised or grown are generally not in the control of the consumer, when eating out, although some restaurants will accommodate special needs, if requested. Generally speaking, this means that in order to follow a healthy food plan that becomes a permanent lifestyle habit, most meals will need to be prepared at home.

As consumers, we prefer what is least expensive, but we need to consider why the cost of a food product is low. Our industrialized food supply, designed to provide large volumes of inexpensive food, is ultimately costing the American population its health. Common animal husbandry practices include providing antibiotics to animals, as well as feeding them grains or other foods that they would not normally eat, to encourage accelerated growth of the animals for increased profit. While this may seem like a great opportunity for the producer, it leaves low levels of antibiotic residue in our food products, potentially disrupting the microbial flora of our gastrointestinal tracts. It also switches the fatty acid composition of our meats to include more pro-inflammatory omega-6 fatty acids, over the anti-inflammatory omega-3 fatty acids. The result is that it tends to tip the body's scale to favor inflammation. It is for this reason that we encourage consumption of organic grass-fed, pastured or free-range and wild-caught animals, including game and cold water fatty fish.

Go organic with your fruits and vegetables. Pesticides on conventionally grown crops are known endocrine disruptors and are toxic to the neurological system. Endocrine disruptors have the capability to influence hormonal systems such as estrogen, thyroid, and neurotransmitter systems[55]. This can affect our capacity to reproduce, develop and grow, or deal with stress and other challenges. Pesticides are in widespread use in our conventional food supply and are not limited to Genetically Modified Food Products (GMOs). These include atrazine, methoxychlor, vinclozolin, prochloraz, and dieldrin. This is not to mention industrial contaminants that find their way into our food supply, such as cadmium and mercury. It is for this reason that certified organic produce is the gold standard. If you know of a local producer that you trust, that grows food with sustainable agricultural practices or integrated pest management and does not use pesticides, but also does not have that organic food label, this is a close equivalent. If your budget only allows for a certain amount of organic food, become familiar with The Dirty Dozen as the top conventionally grown foods to avoid.

Another important strategy is to gravitate toward local food. This is for a variety of reasons. If you know where your food comes from, you will be able to make better food choices. While some of the foods that are recommended in this guide can be purchased at the local grocery store chain, many can also be purchased at local farmers' markets, where they may also be less expensive.

Building relationships with local producers is a great way to secure local foods. Some local producers do not frequent local farmers' markets because of the expense of being a vendor at the markets. Have you ever seen a sign on the side of the road, advertising eggs for sale? Don't be afraid to stop and check it out. Take notice of the farmer's animal husbandry practices. Are the chickens running free range, with access to plenty of bugs and grass, or are they hemmed up in close quarters? What types of feeds and supplements have they been given? Non-GMO and organic would be best. A similar quality of egg may be found at the grocery store for double the cost.

Whether cows grazing on grass, pigs in a pasture or chickens free ranging in a yard, these are all-natural environments for these animals. When animals and plants are raised in their natural environments, they also retain many health benefits from the nutrients available in these surroundings. The effects of sunshine, plenty of space, strong soil and the nutrition in fresh green grass cannot be replicated by the "enrichments" in synthetic feeds. Local fruits and vegetables can be picked at the peak of ripeness, rather than shipped half way across the country to ripen on the way, making them thousands of miles fresher and better for you. So, head to the local farmers' market, and when shopping, don't be afraid to ask questions or try a new vegetable. Be adventurous with your food!

The subject of Increased Intestinal Permeability or "leaky gut," and its relationship to brain health was discussed in **Part 1** of this book. In our clinic we assume that most of us, to some degree, have leaky guts. Nutrient imbalances, food additives, infections, toxic elements or chemical exposures (including those from medications), gut microbial imbalance, excessive oxidative stress, excessive alcohol consumption, direct tissue trauma, electromagnetic radiation, and emotional stress can all cause inflammation and contribute to Leaky Gut Syndrome. The frontline of defense to heal a leaky gut is removing the foods and other offending agents that are causing the increased intestinal permeability in the first place, while replacing them with anti-inflammatory and healing nutrients. This is where we will start our new food adventure.

The cornerstone of *The Brain Tune Up! Food and Recipe Guide* is the popular "Five R's" approach, as taught by The Institute for Functional Medicine. It is part of what would also be called an Elimination Diet. It encourages consumption of a wide variety of foods that are known to be anti-inflammatory to the human system, while eliminating those that commonly trigger food sensitivities or allergies. The foods that are eliminated are sugar, soy, gluten-containing grains, dairy, corn, peanuts, and meats that are processed or come from farms where the animals are raised in unnatural environments (like feedlots and fish farms). This includes typical store-bought beef, and fish such as Atlantic salmon or tilapia.

Here is a summary of **The 5 R's** (more later):

Remove – Any foods, chemicals, or medications that may be causing inflammation, disruptions to the microbes in the digestive tract, and "leakiness" of the gut epithelium.

Replace – With anti-inflammatory foods and additional supplements, if necessary, for digestion (such as enzymes, betaine HCl, bile salts).

Re-inoculate – With prebiotics and probiotics. *Prebiotics* are foods that support gut bacteria and *probiotics* are the beneficial microorganisms that help to maintain and defend gut integrity.

Repair – By providing key micronutrients to help heal the gut.

Rebalance – By addressing lifestyle issues, which also affect the gastrointestinal tract, such as sleep, exercise, food choices, and stressors. Evaluate old habits, so as not to fall back on them.

What are anti-inflammatory foods? Anti-inflammatory foods are first-and-foremost represented by a well-balanced diet. This is a diet in which all the nutrients your body needs are represented in optimal quantities, and consumed by you as real, whole food — the kind of food that does not need a label to tell you what it is. This is the kind of food that has a mother or comes from the earth, using best animal husbandry and good agricultural practices. Reflected in this statement is the concept of *food synergy* or the idea that whole food has superior effects on the body, compared to isolated constituents (like taking supplement vitamins or minerals). Food is information for the body, and those who subscribe to the concept of food synergy believe that this information is best delivered in its natural state. Our cells are evolved to recognize food over isolated components and assimilate the informational and life-sustaining value of food when it is presented in this way.

There are several essential nutrients, meaning nutrients your body cannot synthesize on its own. These include sufficient carbohydrate consumption (even on a low carbohydrate diet), adequate high-quality protein, and fats. Protein is made up of building blocks called amino acids, and among the 20 amino acids needed for life, nine are considered "essential." This is because the body cannot manufacture them on its own. The essential amino acids are histidine, isoleucine, leucine, lysine, methionine, phenylalanine, threonine, tryptophan, and valine. Proteins are needed for tissue structure (like muscle), enzyme production, and neurotransmitter synthesis. Fats have been given a bad rap since Ancel Keys released his *Seven Countries Study*, which influenced food policy for decades. He was an American physiologist who studied the influence of diet on health and hypothesized that saturated fat causes cardiovascular heart disease. The government bought that argument. The low-fat trend that followed is likely a major contributor to the obesity and diabetes epidemic facing this country, and to many conditions that affect the brain, which, by the way, is mostly made of fat!

Fats play a crucial role in energy storage and production, are an integral component of all cell membranes, are essential for the absorption of certain vitamins (A, D, E, and K), and are necessary for hormone synthesis. Taking the food synergy concept further, we should ideally strive for all the vitamins and minerals our bodies need to be acquired through food. In a proper anti-inflammatory diet, then, this means eating enough food. By recommending the right kinds of food with an awareness of meeting their nutrient needs, our patients frequently lose weight, even without counting calories. Furthermore, they see improvements in blood pressure, cholesterol, insulin and blood sugar levels, and many successfully wean off medications that they have been taking to control these measures. All of this benefits the aging brain.

Finally, anti-inflammatory diets are rich in phytonutrients. This class of micronutrients (the other classes are vitamins and minerals) comes exclusively from plants and consists of thousands of chemicals with remarkable health-promoting properties. A few examples of phytonutrients include carotenoids, flavonoids, and ellagic acid. Carotenoids are responsible for the colors of vegetables and fruits — yellow, orange, and red. We are all familiar with the orange carotenoids, alpha- and beta-carotene, found in pumpkin and carrots. Lycopenes give tomatoes and watermelon their red or pink color. Ellagic acid is found in berries, such as strawberries and raspberries. Flavonoids include the catechins of green tea, and the flavonols, such as quercetin in apples. These phytonutrients have diverse capabilities, including their roles in fighting off cancer, antioxidant, and anti-inflammatory benefits.

While an anti-inflammatory diet emphasizes consumption of large amounts of green leafy vegetables, cruciferous sulfur-producing vegetables (such as broccoli, cauliflower, and cabbage), colorful vegetables, and low-sugar fruits such as berries, our anti-inflammatory diet is not, per se, a vegetarian diet. Well-sourced animal-based food delivers certain nutrients that cannot be derived from plants. These include the omega 3 fatty acids DHA (docosahexaenoic Acid) and EPA (Eicosapentaenoic Acid), vitamin B12 (critical for a healthy nervous system), creatine (energy for muscles), carnosine (an antioxidant), taurine (which plays a role in muscle function, bile salt formation, and the body's antioxidant defense system), vitamin D3 (necessary for proper immune function, while deficiency is associated Alzheimer's, multiple sclerosis, and depression) and heme-iron (an excellent source of iron from meat).

In the final analysis, this a diet designed to optimally feed your brain. The goal is to provide your brain with the nutrients it needs to prevent memory loss and protect this critical organ from what is too often attributed to "normal" aging. When, in your mid-50's, for example, you cannot remember the names of friends you have known for years, it is not normal aging. To give your brain a tune up, your diet needs to be sufficiently nutrient-dense to support moment-to-moment operations. This is food-as-information. It not only means adequate carbohydrates, protein, and healthy fats, but fat-soluble vitamins (A, D, and E), B-vitamins, antioxidants (including vitamin C and alpha lipoic acid), and minerals, such as magnesium and zinc. To be clear, there is an emphasis on food synergy in this plan. We want you to get as many of the nutrients your brain needs to function optimally from the food that you eat. Green leafy vegetables such as kale, collards, spinach, watercress and Swiss chard are high in A, C, and fiber. Fiber-containing foods also support gut bacteria, which produce short-chain fatty acids like butyrate, energy for your brain. Just one serving a day of green leafy vegetables has been shown to slow cognitive decline.

The reason you are asked to eat lots of sulfur rich foods such as garlic, mushrooms and onions as well as cruciferous vegetables such as broccoli, cauliflower, Brussels sprouts, kale and cabbage is because of the essential role they play in supporting glutathione production, one of your body's main antioxidant and detoxification molecules. You will notice that the recipes are loaded with these types of foods. You may even wish to consider organ meat, such as chicken liver, because it is an excellent source of B vitamins (B12, B6 and folate, in particular), Vitamin A, and iron. Another potent antioxidant, alpha lipoic acid, is also found in organ meats as well as spinach, broccoli, peas and tomatoes. Alpha lipoic acid is important because it helps your body to recycle vitamin C and supports glutathione production, as well. This is one of the many reasons we encourage you to "eat your colors." In general, the foods high in antioxidants are also very colorful, so eat plenty of blueberries, strawberries, sweet potato and red cabbage, to name few.

The minerals magnesium and zinc, discussed in detail in the supplement chapter of this book, are still best obtained, where possible, from food. Magnesium can be found in green leafy vegetables, avocados, nuts, and legumes, while zinc is found in grass-fed meats, nuts, and seeds. Nuts, oils, green leafy vegetables and avocado tend to be the highest sources of vitamin E. Shellfish, like oysters, mussels and clams, are rich in B-vitamins, zinc, and selenium. As you can see, no one food or food group provides just one vitamin or mineral. We lean heavily toward plant-based foods with a modest portion of meat to provide nutrients you cannot get from an exclusively plant-based diet. This is the reason that we encourage a wide variety of foods within all food groups, and want you to venture beyond the recipes provided, to enjoy the different tastes and flavors offered by these highly nutritious, brain-supporting foods.

You may find it difficult to understand why you are being asked to eliminate certain foods from your diet. Let me explain. First, the foods that are eliminated are those that tend to trigger food allergies or food sensitivity reactions, most commonly. Gluten, a mixture of two proteins, glutenin and gliadin, is naturally found in wheat and certain other grains, and is responsible for the elasticity of dough. Celiac disease is an autoimmune condition which occurs in those with a specific genetic predisposition, and it destroys the surface lining of the small intestine, when gluten is consumed. In the process, the intestinal barrier is disrupted. Symptoms of Celiac disease include pain, diarrhea, nausea, vomiting, maldigestion, and other long term systemic effects, if left unaddressed. Of course, most people do not have Celiac disease. But it is clear that a substantial proportion of people remain sensitive to gluten, and some may test positive for autoimmune reactivity, even without having obvious digestive symptoms.

Gluten reactivity in the central nervous system implies inflammation and a "leaky brain." The spectrum of gluten-related neurological symptoms can include psychiatric disorders from bipolar disorder and depression to schizophrenia and attention deficit disorder. Gluten can trigger brain fog, migraines, sleep disturbance, seizures, and uncoordinated arm and leg movements. Effects reported outside of the central nervous system include peripheral nerve disease and inflammatory muscle disease. In fact, according to one study, patients with neurological diseases of unknown cause were found to have a much higher prevalence of circulating antibodies to gluten (57%) in their blood than either controls (12%) or those with neurological disorders of known cause (5%)[56].

Other foods may cross-react with gluten so that your body may think you are still eating gluten: in particular, dairy, corn, and soy. The casein proteins in the dairy are thought to be cross-reactive (less commonly, whey). Corn and soy are genetically modified crops. Genetic modifications allow industrial farmers to apply poisons such as glyphosate to a crop, to kill weeds while not damaging the food crop itself, and in the case of corn, another genetic modification causes the corn to produce a toxin (Bt) that kills corn-eating caterpillars. In 2011, Canadian researchers found Bt residues in the blood of mothers and fetuses, despite claims of safety to human populations.[57] Glyphosate has been declared a "probable carcinogen" by the World Health Organization and the State of California has also listed it as carcinogenic. Symptoms of corn allergy can include gastrointestinal distress and headaches.

Like corn, most soy is genetically modified in order to make it resistant to herbicides, including glyphosate. For individuals who are not sensitive to soy, or who have no identifiable immunological cross-reactivity, non-GMO soy, particularly, fermented soy foods (natto, tempeh, and miso), may be considered for reintroduction after the initial phase of this *Healthy Brain Toolbox* diet.

Eggs, while a common allergy-causing food, are an excellent source of protein, healthy fat and fat-soluble vitamins, particularly when acquired from chickens that are pastured, free-ranging, and eating seeds and insects. Although eggs are eliminated initially, to give your digestive tract the most optimal stimulus for healing, they should be a top candidate for later re-introduction. Shellfish, such as oysters, clams, mussels, and scallops are removed initially, for the same reason as eggs, but they are outstanding sources of B-vitamins and minerals, and can, for many people, be safely reinstated as individual foods are explored over time.

Perhaps the biggest culprit is sugar. The impact of sugar has already been discussed in **Part 1**. This discussion of sugar includes all foods considered to be refined carbohydrates or high on the <u>glycemic index or glycemic load</u>. This means that the body readily turns these food products into sugar, regardless of their form. The metabolic impacts of a high sugar diet are diverse, and are associated with obesity, diabetes, and the risk of Alzheimer's disease. Sugar forms those advanced glycation end-products that damage multiple components of cells, including DNA, increase oxidative stress and inflammation, and fuel the growth of cancers. This is why foods high in carbohydrate, regardless of source, are limited on this meal plan, at the outset.

If you are ready to make changes in your diet to protect your aging brain, here are some steps you can take to set yourself up for success:

Involve your family or support network. Sit down and have a discussion about why you are doing what you are doing and invite them to be part of these dietary changes to protect your brain. Do not be afraid to discuss this with close, supportive friends, as well. The more support you have, the more successful you are likely to be.

Plan ahead. Any new habit you start will require some advanced planning. Gather your grocery list, chop vegetables in advance, and prep for a few days, not just one day.

Find ways to enjoy the change. Cook with friends and family, listen to music while cooking, create new recipes, try some new foods (preferably on your list of foods okay to eat), or consider growing some of your own food. There is something fundamentally rewarding about planting and growing your own food. A fresh herb garden in the kitchen window is easy to maintain, and fresh herbs taste so much better!

Buy some great kitchen utensils. If you don't already have some of these, I recommend a salad spinner, microplane, crock-pot, and a hearty blender (Ninja® or Vitamix®). Use a good knife! When you have a good, sharp knife, cutting up those vegetables is more enjoyable. Consider finding glass or stainless steel containers as way to store food in your refrigerator, rather than plastic. Most plastics contain bisphenol-A, which is an endocrine disruptor.

Ask yourself, "What are my barriers to success?" Be realistic, and purposefully work toward breaking those barriers down. Do you find cooking stressful? Ask yourself what you find stressful about it and develop a game plan to address this issue. Do you feel you are too busy to cook? Most of these recipes take less than 30 minutes, as long as the prep work has been done in advance. Notice your eating patterns. Do you tend to eat on the fly? Are you an emotional eater? Purposefully identify what keeps you from making healthier food choices and actively develop a plan to manage it.

Get a journal. Write down your goals and your action plan to achieve those goals. Track your progress in your journal. Or use an app to track progress. One company, called <u>Self Care Catalysts</u>, has an app called Neuro Health Storylines® available for <u>Android</u> and <u>iOS</u> devices. Whether you track on paper or in digital form, you can go back and objectively look at your success over the long and short term.

Let's Begin!

The approach to nutrition — in our office and in this book — is designed to settle down the inflammation by removing foods that can cause it. Following are the guidelines for the Start Up phase. The more closely you follow the Start Up plan, the more successful you will be in settling down inflammation. Remember, too, that this is not just for your gut; it is for your brain. The healthier your digestive tract, the better you will feel, and you will have taken an essential step to protect your aging brain. In the Start Up phase:

There are no calorie limits. We want you to eat until you are almost full, but not overeat. It helps to eat until you are 80-90 percent full, then take a short break, and let your satiety hormones catch up. You may find after a few minutes that you feel you have eaten enough. If not, eat a little more. This is about getting all the nutrients your body needs, and your body will let you know.

Use only the foods on the lists.

Do not be afraid to add snacks into your meal plan, if you are hungry between meals. We have included some ideas for snacks, in the menu section.

Choose organic whenever possible. This goes for all meats, fruits and vegetables, as well as allowed grains. If you are worried about the cost, do not eat out! Avoiding restaurants will prevent you from eating unhealthy food and save you money.

Eat at least 9 servings of fruits and vegetables daily. (This may sound like a lot, but watch how easy this is!) Serving size is one cup if raw, ½ cup if cooked. Limit fruits to 1-2 servings per day.

Simple foods are best. If a food has more than 5-6 ingredients on the label, and you do not recognize the ingredients as food, it's probably not a good choice. Avoid food additives and preservatives, as these may also cause inflammation and damage the intestinal microbiome.

If you know you have a specific food sensitivity or allergy, avoid it, even if allowed in this meal plan.

Fast 12 hours overnight. Wait 12 hours between your evening meal and breakfast the next morning. No eating for several hours before bedtime is ideal. You will rest better.

No more than 6 servings of high carbohydrate foods per day. This is to limit your glycemic response to foods. High carb foods in this plan include fruit, non-gluten-containing grains, and starchy vegetables. (See list in "Retain" section.)

Two-thirds of your plate should be vegetables or plant-based foods. Meat should be the smallest portion (about the size of the palm of your hand), and the rest of your plate should be full of color.

Have fun with your food. I know your mother told you not to play with your food, but the more you enjoy working with food in the kitchen, the more fun you will have, and the more successful you will be with this meal plan. (No food fights, please!)

The 5 R's in more detail:

REMOVE – This is the first R!

Remove dairy, grains containing gluten (wheat, barley, and rye), corn, soy, table sugar, artificial sweeteners, shellfish, pork, peanuts, processed meats, grain-fed, industrially raised or factory farmed meats, convenience foods, and alcohol from your diet. (Alcohol for cooking is an exception.) For many, this will mean removing the majority of the foods that you eat. Rest assured that there are still plenty of wholesome, delicious foods that are allowed.

REPLACE – This is the second R!

Replace those foods with the following:

CHOOSE – grass-fed, organic beef, lamb or bison. Grass-fed is higher in omega-3s.

CHOOSE – free-range, organic chicken or turkey.

CHOOSE – wild caught salmon, sardines, anchovies, mussels, rainbow trout, Atlantic mackerel, and herring (chosen for high omega-3 but low mercury content).

CHOOSE – wild game (deer, turkey).

RETAIN – all fruit, fresh/frozen vegetables, healthy oils (avocado, sesame, olive, coconut, and walnut oils), lean/fresh meats, nuts, seeds, legumes, non-gluten whole grains (such as quinoa, rice or amaranth). Watch out for consuming too many carbohydrate rich foods, such as peas, potatoes, sweet potatoes, fruits, and grains. Choose No more than 2 carbohydrate-rich foods per meal, and only one per meal if you eat snacks and the snacks include carbohydrates. A serving size is ½ cup (15 grams or 1 carbohydrate-rich food). This is important, because many people I see in my office do not have diagnosed diabetes, but they have elevated insulin levels, which can also influence brain health.

INCLUDE – 2 servings of prebiotic vegetables daily. These include cabbage, Brussels sprouts, garlic, cauliflower, broccoli, asparagus, onions, jicama, dark-green, leafy vegetables (kale, spinach, arugula, Swiss chard).

THINK COLOR – When it comes to fruits and vegetables, color also means antioxidants, and antioxidants are what help your body to fight off those free radicals and the oxidative stress that negatively influences your health.

DRINK – at least 8 cups of hydrating beverages daily (herbal tea, water, kombucha). To calculate your own fluid needs, divide your body weight in pounds by 2, and drink that many ounces a day. Example: A 135-pound woman would drink 67.5 ounces a day (a little more than half a gallon). Please don't limit yourself to this as a standard. If you are working out or beginning to work out as part of your healthy lifestyle change, your fluid needs will be higher, and you will need to replace the fluids you lose through sweat. Replace 16 ounces for every pound lost during exercise.

USE – only natural sugars to sweeten in recipes. These include maple syrup, honey, stevia and coconut sugar, but no more than 3-4 tsp per day.

RE-INOCULATE – This is the third R!

ADD – a probiotic blend (25 to 50 CFU) with *lactobacillus* and *bifidobacterium*, and fermented (live cultured) foods such as kimchi, sauerkraut, kombucha, coconut kefir or coconut yogurt — 1 to 2 half-cup servings per day, every day. Think of your intestinal tract as the forest floor after a wildfire has gone through and decimated all the undergrowth below the larger oaks and pines. The reforestation will either be from whatever the wind blows in, or it can be purposefully repopulated with flora and fauna that support the ecosystem.

REPAIR – This is the fourth R!

Start with a natural triglyceride form omega-3 blend of at least 1000 mg of DHA and EPA combined, a high CFU (Colony Forming Units) probiotic, turmeric, and Vitamin D3 at 5,000 IU daily. Make sure the supplements you use have been tested and found to be of pharmaceutical grade quality. Although we want you to get almost all the nutrients you need from food, it is our experience that most people have insufficient levels of omega-3 fatty acids and vitamin D, when they are measured. These supplements help with gut repair.

REBALANCE – This is the fifth R!

Once again, this is where your journal is especially helpful. When you write down how what you are eating affects your overall well-being, it allows you to make more mindful decisions about food, moving forward. Don't hold back. The more truthful you are on paper, the more insight you will gain, and the greater possibility of long term success. This journal should include entries about sleep, movement and exercise, stress resilience practice, and social interaction. If you are writing down everything, you will know if other aspects of your life need attention. This exercise helps to remind yourself that this rebalancing of habits is about overall brain health, and all these lifestyle factors work best to create that health, if they are integrated together.

Day 1 – Planning

This is your planning day. Take the time to work through what you plan to eat over the next few days. Review the menus. Make sure you are able to eat everything on them. If you have allergies or intolerances to any foods, see if you can find suitable substitutions that still follow the basic guidelines of the food plan. Inventory what you have at the house, and make note of what you need. Consider emptying your cabinets and refrigerator of old or expired food items at this time, as well. Perhaps donate convenience foods to the local food pantry so that in a pinch, you will be less likely to fall back on foods not on the food plan.

It may be necessary to go to more than one market to obtain the food items you need. Be aware of this, and have a backup plan. If you know that the grocery store you usually shop at is not likely to carry organic produce or meats, plan to go to a different market. Advance planning to attend farmers' markets to obtain grass-fed or pasture-raised organic food products will ensure success on your new food adventure. If at all possible, do this with a friend or relative. This not only helps with the stress associated with making major changes, but will give you one more opportunity to strengthen your relationships with people you love and care about. Prepare food in advance whenever possible.

Develop a game plan to drink an appropriate amount of fluids. Some people are unaware that they do not drink enough, and never get thirsty. After calculating your needs, as previously mentioned in the "Guidelines" section, grab your favorite cup and decide how many of them you have to drink in a day, to meet your needs. Adequate amounts of fluids are important to brain health, to ensure appropriate hydration, as are bowel habits that facilitate detoxification.

Day 2

A note on salt and flavor: When you make these recipes, please remember that salt and pepper to taste means exactly that. Many people look past this portion as just a side note, but seasoning to a flavor that you enjoy is key to success, as long as you are not eating *too* much salt. If you have a tendency to add a lot of salt to foods, start with the base recipe, taste it and then add a little. Getting back in touch with appreciating the flavor of the food itself, rather than the flavor of salt, is one of the great benefits to cooking at home. Sea salt or Himalayan salt is preferred.

For perspective, one full teaspoon of table salt contains slightly greater than 2300 mg of sodium, which is more than most people need in a day. Unless you are under specific sodium restriction by your doctor's orders, your body should be able to handle the salt in the recipes, as long as you are eating plenty of fruits and vegetables. Some people require more salt because of losses during exercise. This could be one more reason to break a sweat!

Breakfast – Day 2

Kale/Cashew Smoothie

Don't feel like cooking a meal? Start out with blenderized bliss that supports your microbiome as well. Throwing these ingredients in a blender takes less than 5 minutes, and the resulting smoothie is packed with nutrition. (This recipe has 3 carbohydrate-rich foods, so share a little with a friend.)

Ingredients:

- 1 cup kale, stems and all
- ¼ cup cashews
- 1 banana
- 2 scoops pea protein powder (vanilla flavored)
- ½ teaspoon fresh ginger, *minced*
- 1 tsp honey
- 1 cup unsweetened almond milk
- 1 cup ice cubes
- Water to desired thickness

The kale can be switched out with other greens, if you have them available. Clean the greens first, in your salad spinner. Place all ingredients in a blender, and blend until smooth. Add water for desired thickness. Enjoy!

Snack – Day 2

Roasted Almonds

Make your own. Toss raw almonds in a frying pan set on medium heat. Spray with extra light olive oil or avocado oil, salt lightly, and sprinkle on some rosemary.

Lunch – Day 2

Wild-Caught, Pan-Seared Salmon with Mango Salsa

Talk about an anti-inflammatory meal! Your palate and your body will be super invigorated when you are finished with this 30-minute meal. Don't be afraid to make extra salsa and mix it with some black beans for a leftover meal the next day. This is perhaps the most complicated recipe, but you will not be disappointed that you tried this! (This meal has 1 carbohydrate per serving, if you limit yourself to ½ a cup of mango salsa.)

Ingredients:

- 2 ripe mangoes, *peeled, pitted, and diced*
- ¼ medium red onion, *finely chopped*
- ½ red bell pepper, *chopped*
- ½ jalapeno pepper, *seeds removed, finely chopped*
- 3 Tablespoons fresh cilantro, *chopped*
- 1 ½ fresh limes, *divided*
- 3 Tablespoons extra-virgin olive oil, *divided*
- Salt, to taste
- Freshly ground black pepper, to taste
- ½ pound salmon filets
- 1 ripe avocado, *peeled, pitted and sliced*
- 4 big handfuls of mixed spring greens

In a medium sized bowl, combine the mango, red onion, jalapeno, cilantro, and juice from ½ of a lime. Set aside. In a small bowl, make a salad dressing by whisking together 2 tablespoons of the olive oil, the juice from another ½ a lime, a pinch of salt, and few grinds of black pepper. Set aside.

Cut the salmon into 2 equal pieces. Take note of any bones in the meat and use a clean pair of tweezers to remove. Squeeze the juice of the remaining ½ lime over the salmon, and season lightly with salt and black pepper.

Heat the remaining 1 tablespoon of olive oil in a skillet over medium-high heat. Put the salmon into the pan, skin-side-down, and cook until the flesh of the fish turns opaque about ⅓ of the way up the side, usually 3 to 5 minutes. Turn it over and sear the second side until it is just cooked through, another 3 to 5 minutes, depending on the thickness of the filets. When fully cooked, the fish will easily flake with a fork.

Dress the greens with the olive oil/lime juice dressing. Arrange the greens and the mango salsa along with the salmon. Serve.

Snack – Day 2

Pear or **apple:** If the size of a tennis ball either of these will count as one carbohydrate-rich food.

Supper – Day 2

Whole Chicken with Rosemary and Garlic

This fantastic recipe will not disappoint you! It is simple and delicious, and leaves lots of leftovers to use in other recipes.

Ingredients:

- 1 free range organic chicken, *whole*
- 4 garlic cloves, *minced*
- 2 sprigs of rosemary, *finely chopped*
- 3-4 Tablespoons grass-fed ghee
- ½ cup dry white wine (Chablis works well.)
- 1 cup white or yellow onion, *sliced thinly*

Set the oven on 350°F. Place chicken on a rack inside a roasting pan. Mix garlic, rosemary and ghee together and spread over the top of the chicken, as well as in the cavity of the chicken. Pour ½ cup dry white wine in the cavity of the chicken. Place onions on the underside of the chicken, where drippings from the chicken will land on them. Cook chicken until its internal temp reaches 165 degrees. This may take up to an hour and half, depending upon the size of the bird. Let chicken rest before serving. Cut desired part of the chicken and serve with the cooked onions over the top.

Classy Quinoa

One of the easiest gluten-free, high-antioxidant grains is not only delicious but also quite versatile. High in quercetin and kaempferol, these antioxidants have been shown to fight inflammation! Here, we double the recipe, to have plenty on hand to use later in the week. (½ cup is the equivalent of one carbohydrate-rich food.)

Ingredients:

- 4 cups bone broth
- 2 cups quinoa (any kind or color)
- Salt and pepper, to taste

Bring the cooking liquid to a boil. (This can be made with water, as well, but the end product will not be as flavorful or as good for you.) Stir in the quinoa, then turn the heat down to low. Cover and simmer until all the liquid is absorbed, about 15 minutes. Use a fork to fluff and separate the grains.

Sautéed Spinach and Mushrooms

Quick, easy and delicious! Remember, mushrooms are your detoxing friends!

Ingredients:

- 3 cups spinach, *washed*
- 2 Tablespoons olive oil or grass-fed ghee
- 1 cup mushrooms, *washed and diced*
- 1-2 garlic cloves, *minced*
- Salt and pepper, *to taste*

Heat olive oil or ghee in skillet on medium-low to medium heat. Add mushrooms and garlic, and sauté until mushrooms begin to brown. Add spinach and stir until spinach begins to reduce. Reducing the spinach usually only takes a few minutes. Salt and pepper, to taste. Serve!

Kale Salad

This salad is so easy to make, and so delicious. Even people who don't like kale love this salad! (Cranberries are the carbs. 1 ½ tablespoons is one carb.) Count your serving of this salad as one carbohydrate-rich food.

Ingredients:

- One bunch of curly leaf or purple kale
- ¼ cup olive oil
- 1 teaspoon lemon juice
- 1 Tablespoon apple cider vinegar
- 1 Tablespoon agave nectar
- ¼ teaspoon salt
- ¼ cup dried cranberries or other dried fruit
- ¼ – ½ cup toasted pumpkin seeds

Separate the kale leaves from their stems by taking the top of a stem and running your other hand down from the thickest part of the stem to the smallest, to remove the leaves. This technique literally takes seconds, to prepare the kale. You can also use pre-packaged, pre-cut organic kale. Break apart into smaller 1 to 2-inch square pieces, then rinse completely in a salad spinner. Place in a bowl.

Mix the olive oil, lemon juice, apple cider vinegar, salt, and agave nectar together well, and then pour over the kale. Massage it into the kale with your fingers until most of the leaves are covered. Toss the cranberries and seeds on top before serving.

Day 3

Breakfast – Day 3

AM Quinoa Bowl

An unusual addition to the breakfast meal, we eat this any time of day and just call it something different. In the morning, a farm fresh sunny side up egg is added, to call it breakfast! (Note: Eggs should be removed during Phase 1, but may be reintroduced after the first month.) This recipe is also packed with tons of antioxidant additions! (1 cup is one carbohydrate-rich food.)

Ingredients:
- 2 cups cooked quinoa
- 2 farm fresh organic eggs (optional, after Phase 1 is completed)
- 2 Tablespoons olive oil or coconut oil
- ½ cup yellow onions or scallions, *diced*
- ½ cup carrots, *diced*
- 1 cup kale, *cut into approximately 1-inch pieces*

- 1 garlic clove, *minced*
- ½ cup cherry or grape tomatoes, *cut in half*
- ½ pound grass-fed ground lamb (This can be done with other meats, as well.)
- Salt and pepper, *to taste*

Pour oil into a warm skillet. Add onion and carrots, and sauté until onion is beginning to turn brown. Then add garlic, tomatoes and kale. Sauté until kale begins to break down. Remove from skillet and set aside, covered to retain heat.

Begin browning the lamb in the same skillet. At the same time, in a separate skillet, begin cooking eggs (if using) in olive oil. Flip when eggs will not fall apart, and make sure the yolks are cooked well. This only takes a few minutes on either side, with a hot skillet. After lamb has been browned and cooked thoroughly, add vegetables to the same skillet to rewarm and mix together. Take approximately 1 cup of the mixture, place in a bowl with one egg (if using) on top and serve!

Snack – Day 3

¼ – ½ cup trail mix (This may be 1 carb, depending on how much dried fruit is in your serving. Two tablespoons = one carbohydrate-rich food.)

Trail Mix

Make a batch of this and have it available at your desk at work or at home. If raw foods are not tolerated, it is okay to purchase the roasted versions of the nuts or buy raw nuts and roast them yourself in an oven. Don't be afraid to use different nuts and dried fruits, based on preference.

Ingredients:

- ¼ cup almonds (raw, organic)
- ¼ cup walnuts (raw, organic)
- ¼ cup hazelnuts (raw, organic)
- ¼ cup cashews (raw, organic)
- 3 Tablespoons pumpkin seeds (raw, organic)
- 2 Tablespoons sunflower seeds (raw, organic)
- 3 Tablespoons organic raisins (dark or golden)
- 3 Tablespoons organic dried cranberries (no sugar added)
- 2 Tablespoons dried goji berries (These add a nice crunch to your mix, and they are antioxidant rich.)
- ¼ tsp <u>unrefined sea salt</u>

Mix all ingredients in a medium-sized mixing bowl. Transfer to a quart-sized baggie or glass container.

Lunch – Day 3

Organic Herb-Roasted Turkey Breast

This can be made in advance, and then reheated for a quick and easy lunchtime meal.

Ingredients

- 1 bone-in turkey breast
- 1 Tablespoon olive oil
- 1-2 teaspoons black pepper
- 1 teaspoon dried rosemary
- 1 teaspoon dried thyme
- 1 teaspoon garlic salt
- 1 medium onion, *cut into wedges*
- ½ cup white wine or chicken broth

Preheat oven to 325 degrees. Brush olive oil all over the skin of the turkey. Then combine rosemary, thyme, and garlic salt, and rub all over turkey. Place onion and celery in a 3-quart baking dish, top with turkey, skin side up, and pour wine into the dish. Bake uncovered for 2 to 2 ½ hours, or until thermometer reads 170 degrees. Baste the turkey periodically with the drippings in the bottom of the pan. Let cool, carve, and serve!

Awesome Quick Brown Lentils

This higher fiber recipe with plenty of extra goodies will make you smile at how easy it is to make! Total cook time is less than 15 minutes. Double the recipe, and have plenty of leftovers for the rest of the week! (½ cup is one carbohydrate-rich food.)

Ingredients:

- 1 Tablespoon olive oil
- 1 cup onion, *chopped*
- ½ cup celery, *diced*
- ½ cup carrots, *diced*
- 1 clove garlic, *minced*
- 2 cups pre-cooked lentils
- Salt and fresh ground pepper, *to taste*

In a large skillet, over medium heat, warm oil and then add onion, celery, and carrot, and cook until soft. Stir in garlic until fragrant. Stir in lentils, and season to taste!

Basic Lentil Recipe

Make this recipe in advance and have on hand to add to the Awesome Quick Brown Lentils or be creative.

Ingredients:

- 4 quarts of water (or preferably, homemade broth)
- 1 pound of brown lentils (rinsed and debris from packaging removed)

Bring 4 quarts of water to a boil. Add 1 pound of lentils. Reduce heat and simmer, uncovered, for 15-20 minutes or until lentils are the desired tenderness. Drain well, allow to cool, and refrigerate or add to other recipes!

Asparagus

Asparagus is super quick and easy to prepare and is a fantastic prebiotic! Like avocados, it is also a great source of glutathione.

Ingredients

- Asparagus
- 1-2 Tablespoons olive oil
- Salt, *to taste*
- ½ lemon

Rinse asparagus and break off any extra fibrous ends. To do this, hold each end of the asparagus and bend gently. The asparagus will break at the point that the tough end changes to tender and edible. Discard the thicker, pale end. Heat oil in skillet on medium-low to medium heat. Place the asparagus in the warm skillet and cook for 2 to 3 minutes. (Should still be crisp.) Squeeze lemon over asparagus and salt to taste, then serve.

Snack – Day 3

Apple or **pear** – whichever you didn't eat yesterday. (This counts as one carbohydrate-rich food.)

Supper – Day 3

Grass-fed Steak

Please read <u>this link</u> before cooking any grass-fed steak. There is an art to cooking grass-fed steaks, and if cooked too long, they can become very rubbery and hard to eat. Most grass-fed products will come frozen, so plan some additional time for thawing.

Ingredients

- Grass-fed T- bone steak, *thawed*
- 1 Tablespoon olive oil
- ½ Tablespoon rosemary, *chopped*
- ½ Tablespoon garlic, *minced*
- Salt and pepper, *to taste*
- Olive oil, to taste

Pat the steak dry with paper towels, then add rosemary and garlic to the top, and cover with cling wrap for at least an hour before cooking. This can be done at room temperature, on a countertop. Follow the directions on the link and serve with the rest of your meal. Feel free to drizzle some olive oil over your steak, if you have never tried this. It is delicious!

Sautéed Button Mushrooms

Mushrooms are a profound detoxifying food. If you are a mushroom fan, this is perhaps one of the easiest recipes we have. Sometimes simple is better!

Ingredients:

- 1 package button mushrooms, *washed*
- 2 Tablespoons olive oil
- 1 Tablespoon balsamic vinegar
- Salt, *to taste*

Heat olive oil in skillet, on medium-low to medium heat. Place whole mushrooms in warm skillet and stir them periodically to ensure that they do not burn. When the mushrooms are fully cooked, add balsamic vinegar and salt to taste! These make a fantastic side to almost any meat dish. Here, we pair with grass-fed steak (above).

Roasted Sweet Potato

Use this recipe with orange or purple sweet potatoes. Remember that this is one of your high carb food servings. (This is potentially 2 carbs, depending on the size of your potato. Approximately ½ cup is one carbohydrate-rich food. Watch the serving size!)

Ingredients:

- 2 sweet potatoes (one for a friend!)
- 1-2 Tablespoons grass-fed ghee or olive oil
- Salt and pepper, to taste

Preheat oven to 400°F. Wrap sweet potatoes individually in tin foil and place in the preheated oven. Cook for 30-45 minutes. Cook time will depend on size and shape of the potato. Remove tin foil. Slice potato lengthwise and add ghee or olive oil. Salt and pepper, to taste!

Brassy Brussels

This recipe was named for its presence in the beloved brassica/cruciferous vegetable family (so important as a prebiotic food, for a healthy gut and healthy brain).

Ingredients:

- 3 cups fresh Brussels sprouts, *thinly sliced*
- ½ cup onion, *thinly sliced and chopped*
- 3 garlic cloves, *peeled and minced*
- 2-3 Tablespoons of either ghee or coconut oil
- Salt and pepper, *to taste*

Heat oil or ghee in skillet on medium heat. Place all ingredients in a warm skillet, stirring occasionally until the onions have begun to turn slightly brown. Salt and pepper, to taste. This recipe is great with a little pork, when added back into the diet, as well.

Day 4

Breakfast – Day 4

Beet/Coconut Smoothie

Not only does this smoothie look pretty and taste great, but it is so good for you! This is an antioxidant powerhouse! (1 ½ carbohydrate-rich foods, if drinking the whole smoothie.)

Ingredients:

- 1 whole beet, greens and all, *rinsed and chopped*
- ½ teaspoon fresh ginger
- ½ cup coconut milk
- ½ cup of berries
- ½ cup raw pineapple
- ¼ cup roasted almonds
- ½ teaspoon vanilla
- 1 tsp honey
- 1 tsp cinnamon
- 1 cup ice cubes

Place all ingredients in a blender, and blend until smooth. This may take a few minutes. Add water as necessary, for desired thickness. Transfer to a cup and enjoy!

Snack – Day 4

Honey Walnuts

This recipe can be made with any nut, and if desired, you can add other spices, relative to your own taste, such as allspice or nutmeg. We offer walnuts, as they are higher in omega-3s! (½ cup is one carbohydrate-rich food.)

Ingredients:

- 1 cup raw walnut halves
- 1 teaspoon ground cinnamon
- 2 Tablespoons raw, organic honey
- 1 pinch of salt

Preheat oven to 350°F. Line a baking sheet with parchment paper and set aside. In a bowl, combine honey, ground cinnamon and salt. Add in walnuts and toss to combine. Spread nuts in single layer on prepared baking sheet. Bake, stirring occasionally, until toasted, about 15-20 minutes. Let cool completely before serving.

Lunch – Day 4

Chicken Salad on a Bed of Mixed Greens

This is perhaps our most labor-intensive recipe, because the chicken meat has to be removed from the bones of the chicken, but after you do this, you can make some bone broth from what is left. Use any parts of the meat that you would like. There are no rules. If you like the dark meat, use the dark meat. It is actually higher in many micronutrients than the light meat, but some people don't like the stronger flavor, so go with your personal preference.

Ingredients:

- 2 cups of chicken, *diced*
- ½ cup onion, *diced*
- ½ cup celery, *diced*
- ½ cup olive oil mayonnaise
- ¼ teaspoon salt
- ¼ teaspoon pepper
- 1 sprig fresh rosemary, *chopped*
- 1-2 cups mixed greens
- 1 Tablespoon olive oil
- Juice of ½ lime

Mix all ingredients in a medium-sized mixing bowl. Season additionally, to taste. Mix together olive oil and lime, then mix with the greens and place on a plate.

Snack – Day 4

Trail mix and/or leftover cut up **pineapple** (If eating pineapple, you need to count this as 1 carbohydrate-rich food per ½ cup.)

Or, if you have a little extra time on your hands . . . try some guacamole with jicama dippers. (See below.)

Squawking Guac

It's called this because everyone talks about how easy it is to make, and how full it is of those fantastic monounsaturated fats and the glutathione that supports overall health!

Ingredients:

- 2 avocados
- ¼ cup red onion, *chopped*
- 1 teaspoon fresh lemon juice
- 2 Tablespoons cilantro (optional)
- Salt and pepper, *to taste*

Places all ingredients in a bowl and mix together until creamy. This recipe can easily be doubled or tripled if you have friends coming over. I don't recommend making this too far in advance, as the avocado will begin to brown, over time. It literally takes less than five minutes to make!

Jicama Dippers

This veggie gets lost in the shuffle behind its better-known prebiotic counterparts, cabbage and Brussels sprouts. High in fiber, it is more commonly seen as a side to seaweed salad in sushi restaurants (½ cup counts as 1 carbohydrate-rich food).

Ingredients:

- 1 jicama, *cut into fries*
- 1 Tablespoon avocado oil
- ¼ teaspoon smoked paprika
- ¼ teaspoon garlic powder
- ¼ teaspoon turmeric
- ¼ teaspoon onion powder
- 1 pinch of cayenne (optional)
- Salt, *to taste*

Preheat oven 400°F. Peel jicama and cut into fries. Bring water to a boil in a medium saucepan on medium heat, add jicama and cook for 8 minutes until jicama is less crunchy. (Skip this step for more crunchy fries.) Drain water, transfer jicama slices to a large bowl, and toss with avocado oil, paprika, garlic, onion, cayenne pepper and sea salt. Place in a single layer on a greased sheet pan. Bake for 30 minutes or until crispy, turning at least once, to ensure uniform baking. Delicious served with Squawking Guac.

Snack-Day 4

Trail mix and/or leftover cut up **pineapple** (If eating pineapple, you need to count this as 1 carb per ½ cup.)

Supper- Day 4

Grass Fed Burger with Rosemary

This easy recipe works well if you only have a few minutes to throw something together, and you still get the benefits of all the omega-3s!

Ingredients:

- 1 pound grass fed beef, *thawed*
- 1 Tablespoon olive oil for the pan
- 1 sprig of rosemary, *chopped finely*
- Salt and pepper, *to taste*

Place hamburger and rosemary in a bowl, and work together with your hands to mix rosemary well with the hamburger. Split the hamburger into 4 separate portions and make patties out of them. Preheat skillet to medium and cook to desired temperature. (Medium to medium-well is what I recommend.)

Wild Rice Blend

This is a fantastic whole grain dish with lots of extras that not only offer pleasing presentation, but added nutritional value. Two-thirds cup of this dish is equal to 1 ½ carbohydrate-rich foods.

Ingredients:

- 2 cups wild rice (or any whole grain rice)
- 4 cups homemade broth
- 1 whole white or yellow onion, *diced*
- 1 carrot, *diced*
- 1 cup mushrooms, *sliced*

- 3 garlic cloves, *chopped finely*
- 2 Tablespoons of olive oil, avocado oil, or coconut oil
- Salt, *to taste*

Place broth and wild rice in a pan and bring to a boil. Reduce temperature and allow rice to simmer until done. For whole grain rice or quinoa, consult the package for cooking times. This can be anywhere from 20-40 minutes.

Meanwhile, preheat skillet to medium, sauté mushrooms, onions, carrot, garlic and olive oil. Cook until onions begin to turn golden brown. Remove from heat, set aside, and cover to retain heat.

When rice is finished, combine onion mixture with rice and salt, to taste. (One serving is ⅔ cup.)

Prebiotic Slaw

Need we say more? Your microbiome will love this!

Ingredients:

- ½ head of purple cabbage, *sliced into thin pieces*
- ½ head of green cabbage, *sliced into thin pieces*
- 1 purple onion, *sliced thin and cut into 1-inch pieces*
- 3 carrots – *sliced into the same size pieces*
- ½ cup Asian Sesame Dressing (See recipe below.)

Mix all ingredients in a large bowl. Add Asian Sesame Dressing. The longer the salad is allowed to set at room temperature, the more the flavors blend together. It actually tastes better, later in the week!

Asian Sesame Dressing

This in an incredible anti-inflammatory dressing to add to your repertoire, with plenty of ginger, garlic and flavor!

Ingredients

- ½ cup extra-virgin olive oil
- 2 Tablespoons balsamic vinegar
- 2 Tablespoons rice vinegar
- 2 Tablespoons coconut amino acids
- 2 cloves garlic, *minced*
- 1 Tablespoon honey (This recipe tastes great without the honey, as well.)
- 1 Tablespoon ginger, *minced*
- 1 teaspoon expeller-pressed sesame oil
- Salt, *to taste*

Microplaning the garlic and ginger allows them to be mixed thoroughly, throughout the dressing. Mix all ingredients together in a bowl well. Pour over salad, or use as dipping sauce, or in coleslaw.

Spinach Salad

So easy, and so packed with nutrition! Substitute strawberries and pecans for carrots and cucumbers, to switch it up a little bit.

Ingredients:

- 4-5 oz. spinach, *rinsed and dried*
- 2 small cucumbers or ½ an English cucumber
- 1 cup grape or cherry tomatoes, *halved*
- 1 medium carrot, *thinly sliced*
- ½ cup red onion, *diced*

Rinse and dry your spinach. Transfer to a large salad bowl. Slice your cucumbers, thinly slice your carrots, and halve your cherry tomatoes. Toss all the veggies into the salad bowl together, and serve with balsamic dressing below.

Basic Balsamic Recipe

Balsamic vinegar is the base for this simple but delicious mixture that you will use over and over again! If possible, make it in advance of use, because the longer it sits, the more the garlic is infused throughout the dressing.

Ingredients:

- ¼ cup balsamic vinegar
- ¼ cup extra virgin olive oil
- 2 cloves of garlic, *peeled and minced*
- ½ teaspoon salt
- ¼ teaspoon pepper, or to taste

In a small bowl, combine all the dressing ingredients. Briskly whisk or shake the dressing ingredients together. Place in container suitable for pouring dressing.

3-Day Shopping List

Fats

Coconut Oil, cold or expeller-pressed (Larger containers are less expensive, per ounce.)

Olive Oil, extra virgin, real (visit www.extravirginity.com or look for California Olive Oil Council Certified (COOC) certified or Extra Virgin Alliance (EVA) on the label – 16 oz.

Sesame Oil, expeller pressed – 8 oz.

Nuts and seeds

Choose raw if you would like to roast yourself or roasted if you want to save some energy for other food projects. These can be purchased less expensively in bulk. (Feel free to buy more to have on hand, as well as any others that you like, but this is all you will need for the next few days.)

Almonds – 8 oz.

Cashews – 8 oz.

Pecans – 8 oz.

Pumpkin Seeds – 8 oz.

Walnuts – 8 oz.

Grains

Lentils (brown) – 1 pound

Whole Grain/Wild Rice blend – 1 pound

Vegetables

Asparagus – 1 bunch

Avocados – 3

Baking Potatoes – 2

Brussels Sprouts – 2 cups or 1 package

Cabbage, 1 head each, both red and green

(These keep well, so don't worry if they seem large.)

Carrots – 4

Celery – ½ cup

Cucumber – 1

Garlic Cloves, fresh – 8 (1-2 heads)

Ginger, whole, fresh

Jalapeno – 1

Kale – 2 bunches or one large bag of cut and chopped

Mushrooms – I package white, 1 package button

Onions – 2 red and 4 white

Red Bell Pepper – 1
Spinach (organic baby) – 1 large bag
Spring Mix – 1 large bag
Sweet potatoes – 2 small
Tomatoes, grape or cherry – 1 package

Fruits
Apple – 1 of any variety
Banana – 1
Berries, any kind you like – 1 cup
Cranberries, dried – 1 package
Goji berries, dried – 1 package
Lemon – 1
Limes – 3
Mangoes – 2
Pear – 1 of any variety
Pineapple, cubed – 1 cup
Raisins – 1 package

Meats/Protein
Beef Steaks, T-bone (grass-fed, organic) – 2
Beef, Ground (grass-fed, organic) – 1 pound
Chicken (pasture-raised, organic) – 1 whole
Eggs (pasture-raised, organic) – 1 dozen (after Phase 1)
Lamb, Ground (grass-fed, organic) – 1 pound
Protein Powder (rice pea blend) – 1 canister
Salmon (wild-caught) – 10 ounces
Turkey Breast (organic) – 1

Spices
Balsamic vinegar – 16 oz.
Cayenne pepper powder

Coconut aminos – 1 bottle
Cilantro – 1 bunch
Garlic powder
Onion powder
Paprika
Rosemary, fresh – 2 sprigs
Vanilla extract

Dairy Substitute
Almond milk – 1 quart carton
Coconut milk – 1 quart carton

Sweetener
Agave nectar – small container

MAINTENANCE

The general guidelines for long-term maintenance were developed with the understanding that while some foods may be able to be tolerated at this juncture, it is possible to re-inflame the gut and brain, and create the same health challenges you had before starting your journey. Long-term, I suggest continuing to omit gluten, dairy, highly processed sugar, and processed foods. (This is the category where most soy, corn and wheat products reside.) If no sensitivity or allergy is identified, eggs may be reintroduced after the first month, then experiment with shellfish, and consider fermented soy products like natto, tempeh, and miso. It is also suggested that organic, non-GMO foods are continued, as well as the foods that are high in pre- and probiotics. Use of alcohol, such as wine, should remain modest and occasional, at most. Hopefully, by this time, you have noticed how much better you feel. Over time, you will notice that your cravings adjust to desire the foods that you have been enjoying most in your new diet lifestyle, rather than the "edible food-like substances" (to borrow from food writer Michael Pollan) that you previously consumed.

You have changed your food environment to include taking charge of meal preparation, and making food a focus, rather than a side note in your daily routine. Starting new habits can be some of the most challenging but also the most rewarding parts of life. Food was meant to nurture health and taste good, and hopefully you see from the recipes provided that it is not only possible, but also desirable for both to be true. If your food tastes good, you will continue to eat it! By sticking with a plant-based diet with lots of color, you can further your journey toward better brain health. Hopefully, you have tracked all the changes that you made, so you can go back and reference where you were then, relative to where you are now. What a difference!

A final word. Everyone's food journey is different. Everyone's health journey is different. But the first steps toward change are essentially the same. If you haven't already, find people to share with, about what you have learned from the changes you've made. You may find that other people have shared similar experiences or have new insights to offer. Building community and support for the changes you have made, and maintenance of your newly established food environment is essential for continued progress. As this chapter ends, the health journey continues. Invite some friends over for some grass-fed steaks and kale salad, to see what to take on next!

CHAPTER 12

To Om and Beyond

An Emotional and Spiritual Stress Resilience Practice Can Improve Your Memory and Grow Your Brain

---

Guest Author: Chuck Renner, OTR, CHT

"The greatest weapon against stress is our ability to choose one thought over the other."

—William James, philosopher

On a metaphysical level, like-minded spirits tend to find one another, in the vastness of the universe. More than 10 years ago, the company that employed me at the time hired <u>Advantage Therapy</u> to provide outpatient rehabilitative services to their patients. Chuck Renner, OTR, CHT, was then — and still is — the owner of Advantage Therapy. I was intrigued by and impressed with the work he and his therapists accomplished with our patients. I know of no other therapist who is so consistently requested by name. Quickly, I realized that Chuck himself is a brand in our community. When in 2015, I decided to open an independent neurology practice with an emphasis on functional medicine, it was an obvious choice to ask Chuck to be part of that vision.

His own journey into non-conventional approaches to healing goes back to about 2004. As he became increasingly disillusioned with how western medicine viewed the management of chronic pain, he began a quest to learn more about how the body, mind, and spirit work together. He studied under many masters, and added notches to his belt as he learned natural and manual therapy techniques to help patients escape the never-ending cycle of pain-depression-fear-anxiety that characterizes those whose lives are trapped in the cave of suffering. Chuck Renner is a master instructor for Primal Reflex Release Technique, and a board member for the Institute of Integrative Pain Management. He has been trained or holds certifications in Augmented Soft Tissue Management, Primal Reflex Technique, Active Release Technique, Muscle Energy Technique, Pain Neutralization Technique, Neurokinetic Therapy, Myokinetic Therapy, Amino Neuro Frequency Therapy, Craniosacral Therapy, Total Motion Release, Emotional Freedom Technique, Mindfulness training, and more. He has been a featured speaker on several occasions, at the annual meeting of the Academy of Integrative Pain Management, where he teaches manual therapy techniques to physicians, to treat low back pain, neck pain, and other body areas that may be affected.

Chuck walks the walk. He believes in exercise and staying active. A husband and father of six grown children and four grandchildren, he enjoys running, hiking, and martial arts. He has advanced black belts in Tenshi Goju Ryu Karate, and he is the Chief Instructor for the Springfield Aikido School. It is an honor to work with Chuck and to consider him a close colleague, and it is a pleasure to present to you his chapter on emotional and spiritual stress resilience practice, the mind-body connection.

Now, please welcome Chuck Renner:

It is difficult to talk about emotional and spiritual stress resilience without first defining the elephant in the room and the reason we need this practice, which is stress itself. According to the American Psychological Association, average stress levels in the U.S. have risen since 2014, from 4.9 to 5.1 on a 10-point stress scale[58]. There has been a particular increase among adults reporting "extreme stress," with 24% saying they were highly stressed in 2015, compared to 18% in 2014. Researchers from Carnegie Mellon University analyzed data from 1983, 2006 and 2009, and found people's self-reported stress levels have increased 10-30% in the last three decades[59].

What is stress? *The Oxford English Dictionary* defines stress as "a state of mental or emotional strain or tension resulting from adverse or demanding circumstances." The word stress comes from the Latin word *strictus*, meaning "tight, compressed, drawn together." Later, this word was translated into Old French as *estrece*, or "narrowness, oppression[60]." Then, finally Old English, around 1300, defines it as *distress*, meaning, "hardship, adversity, force, or pressure." It received its current connotation from Hans Selye, MD, PhD, DSc, FRS, who in 1936 wrote a letter to the editor of *Nature* entitled, "A Syndrome Produced by Diverse Nocuous Agents[61]." Here, he briefly described the basic physical manifestations of stress, divided into three stages. The letter set the stage for his book, *The Stress of Life* (McGraw-Hill 1955), in which he describes stress in terms of his General Adaptation Syndrome. This syndrome is in reaction to stress, and it covers the three stages: (1) Alarm, (2) Resistance, and (3) Exhaustion.

Selye's stages can be explained as follows. In Stage I (Alarm) the body experiences the fight, flight, or freeze response. It is the body's natural reaction to a dangerous situation. Your heart rate will increase, your blood will go to your arms and legs, your adrenal gland will release cortisol (the stress hormone), and you will receive a boost of energy. You can then decide if you will stand and fight, run away, or freeze — literally like a deer in the headlights. This response leads us to Stage

II (Resistance). In this stage, the body will try to repair itself after the stressful event. You will start to calm down, your heart rate and blood pressure will begin to normalize. If the stress is no longer present, you will return to your pre-stress state.

What if the stressful situation is still present? If the stress continues, then your body will stay on alert. This means that cortisol levels will remain higher. Some of the outward signs of this stage would be frustration, irritability and poor concentration. If this state remains, it can lead to the third stage, Stage III (Exhaustion). In this stage, your body is struggling for a long period of time, which can drain you physically and emotionally. You may feel like you want to give up. The physical signs are fatigue, burnout, depression, and anxiety. This stage can weaken your immune system and put you more at risk for stress-related illnesses. In our *Brain Tune Up!* program, we see this on a regular basis, when it comes to many neurological diseases. A search of "psychological stress and multiple sclerosis" in the U.S. National Library of Medicine database, PubMed, yields 395 references relevant to this topic.

To see how stressed out you are, you can go to The HeartMath Institute website, and take a 25 question survey to see if you are stressed out.

"It's not stress that kills us; it is our reaction to it."
—Hans Selye, MD, PhD

The way our bodies and brains physiologically change with stress is well-documented. To see how stress spreads through the body, we need to look at the endocrine system and the Hypothalamic-Pituitary-Adrenal Axis (HPA). Stress, perceived or real, will activate the hypothalamus. This part of the brain connects the endocrine system with the nervous system. When the hypothalamus senses stress, it releases Corticotropin-Releasing Factor (CRF). This stimulates the pituitary gland (the "master gland" that controls all other endocrine glands) to release adrenocorticotropic hormone (ACTH). ACTH, in turn, tells the adrenal glands to release cortisol. If the perceived stress is short-term, then high levels of cortisol in the blood will decrease, and the system will return to a normal, non-stressed state. But chronic, unyielding stress can lead to a disruption in this normal mechanism by desensitizing the axis so the shut off switch does not work.

Sustained stress or over-activation of the HPA axis can lead to the following changes. To the body, it can cause the central nervous system to increase muscle tone and excitability. This constant excitability increases the metabolic rate, which increases blood flow in general, but actual local circulation is diminished by increased muscle tone. This limits oxygen-rich blood to the tissues. In the absence of oxygen, the muscles will use anaerobic respiration for energy production, which leads to increased buildup of lactic acid in the tissues. Then pain-signaling neurotransmitters will be released, and pain can spread to other spinal segments.

In the clinic, what this looks like is someone with muscles that are sore to touch (due to increased lactic acid) and spinal vertebral segments out of alignment (due to increased muscle tone and poor respiration patterns—more chest breathing than diaphragmatic—and poor posture from fatigue). With increased cortisol levels from sustained stress, the impact in the brain is a shrinking effect in the prefrontal cortex[62]. This is an area of the brain responsible for memory and learning. You use the prefrontal cortex to make every day decisions: What to wear? What to plan? It also lets us speak fluently, with meaning. The prefrontal cortex is not the only area affected by sustained high levels of cortisol. It can also lead to a decline in function and volume of the hippocampus. As you can see, chronic levels of stress can have a deleterious effect on the body, brain, and memory.

"When we are no longer able to change a situation, we are challenged to change ourselves."
—Viktor E. Frankl, neurologist, psychiatrist, and author

In this section, I will discuss what you can do to stop this spiral of stress that can have such a negative effect on cognitive function — from memory to planning, from talking to finding where you placed things — to your immune system, hormones, mitochondria, vascular system, joints and biomechanics, and even your digestion, as well as the ability to eliminate toxins from your body. The benefit of meditation has been demonstrated in numerous published studies. Research by Sara Lazar, PhD and her colleagues from Harvard Medical School used MRI to demonstrate that 8 weeks of a Mindfulness-Based Stress Reduction (MBSR) practice is associated with increased cortical thickness of the hippocampus[63] and reduced brain cell volume in the amygdala[64], which is responsible for fear, anxiety, and stress.

In our program, we primarily use two types of meditation or relaxation training. The first is mindfulness meditation. This type of meditation, also known as Mindfulness-Based Stress Reduction, was formally brought into the medical world in 1979 by Jon Kabat-Zinn, PhD. At that time, he recruited chronically ill patients who were not responding to conventional treatments and put them through an 8-week MBSR program. Since that time, numerous studies have been published about the positive effects of mindfulness meditation. "Mindfulness is awareness that arises through paying attention, on purpose, in the present moment, non-judgmentally," says Kabat-Zinn. "It's about knowing what is on your mind."

For this type of meditation or relaxation training, you first need to get into a comfortable position. Make sure the television, radio, and phone are off, the pets are out of the room and you have some space for yourself. Next, begin diaphragmatically breathing. What that means is that you want to see your stomach expand when you breathe in and fall when you breathe out. I think it works best to have a rhythm to your breathing, something like breathe in on a count of 4, pause for a count of 1 and breathe out for a count of 4. You can adjust this rhythm to your own comfortable pace. Then you want to bring your attention to the present moment by focusing on your breath. Concentrate on your breath, feel your stomach rise and fall, feel the oxygen come into your body and your muscles relax as you exhale. Give yourself a few moments to connect to this feeling. Once you have the rhythm down, focus on your breath. Do not try to force thoughts that may wander in and out. When you realize you are distracted, gently focus to bring your attention back to your breath. To help you focus, you can also listen to the sound of your breath. I suggest setting a timer. Try this initially for 5 minutes, twice a day.

Another practice we do is called HeartMath. HeartMath was founded in 1991 by Doc Childre, an internationally renowned expert on stress. Besides founding HeartMath, he is the author of a dozen books on stress, wellness, and heart-based living. He is the creator of the *emWave Stress Relief System*®, which now includes the emWave2 Handheld®, the Inner Balance® (Bluetooth and Lightning versions) for mobile phones, and the emWave2 Professional Systems®.

HeartMath is a system where, with special equipment and sensors, it is possible to measure heart rate variability (HRV), the subtle beat-to-beat variation which occurs in the normally beating heart. Heart Rate Variability is largely determined by the balance between the sympathetic nervous system (sometimes called "Fight or Flight") and the parasympathetic nervous system (sometimes called, "Rest and Digest"). People who tend to have more sympathetic tone also have lower HRV or less beat-to-beat variation, whereas those with more parasympathetic tone tend to have higher HRV or more beat-to-beat variation. Like other things that have been described in this book, balance is optimal. HeartMath, however, takes this further. While it helps to optimize HRV, it also aims to seek maximal coherence. The HeartMath Institute defines coherence as a logical, orderly and harmonious connectedness between parts of a system or between people. Informally, all of us have experienced coherence in social connections when we are sharing ideas with someone with whom we feel connected. Conversely, we always know intuitively when there is no connection.

When folks at The HeartMath Institute discuss heart-rhythm coherence or physiological coherence, they are referring to a specific assessment of the heart's rhythms that appear as smooth, ordered, and sine-wavelike (up and down). From a physics perspective, quoting directly from HeartMath, "When we are in a coherent state, virtually no energy is wasted because our systems are performing optimally, and there is synchronization among various systems in the body, such as the heart, respiratory system, and blood-pressure rhythms, etc." The HeartMath Institute takes this even further, to study the coherence between entire populations around the globe.

The *Brain Tune Up!* program provides each participant who is capable of operating this type of technology an emWave2® handheld device. An exception might be a person with more advanced dementia. The emWave2® can help you make a positive change. This unique training system, with research-based tools and games, helps build inner resilience to more effectively deal with stressful feelings and life's challenges. Five to ten minutes of daily practice can provide greater ease, mental and emotional flexibility, and more positive attitudes, emotions and perspectives. The emWave2® hand held device can be taken anywhere, and is a perfect tool to use to reduce stress and enhance life. You may wish to purchase your own for your healthy brain toolbox.

Something you can try right now is called the Quick Coherence Technique. For this exercise, you do not need anything. It is a two-step process designed by HeartMath. The first step is to slow your breathing and make it heart-centered. This means focus on your heart.

Imagine your breath is flowing in and out of your heart. The second step is to focus on a positive feeling. It could be appreciation for someone; it could be a happy memory; or it could be just a focus on the feeling of calm, peace, serenity, or ease. To start, I recommend people try this for 5 minutes, twice a day.

Rollin McCraty, Director of the HeartMath Institute, refers to coherence as "a state when the heart, mind and emotions are in energetic alignment and cooperation." By mastering the Quick Coherence technique, you have nurtured a state that "builds resiliency, [where] personal energy is accumulated, not wasted," according to McCraty. Then you are ready to take the idea of coherence even further, to use your accumulated energy "to manifest intentions and harmonious outcomes." Recall the case of Eric, from Chapter 1, the business executive with Amyotrophic Lateral Sclerosis. As an outside-the-box thinker, Eric wrote a letter to the consulting neurologist at a major medical center ahead of his visit, asking how he might use lifestyle interventions, including affirmations, to create the proper mindset to heal from his disease. Not surprisingly, he was met with ambivalence, because conventional medicine is largely ill-equipped to address illness with these tools.

What are affirmations? Affirmations are a kind of positive self-talk or talk for the purpose empowerment. The use of affirmations by the conscious mind is a way to program unconscious attitudes, actions, and behaviors so that they are in alignment with our goals. Have you ever heard the expression, "Your words say one thing, but your actions say another?" The idea of affirmations that are repeated and reinforced on a daily basis is to create coherence, not just for moment-to-moment communication, but in the long term. *We become what we say and think.* The remarkable truth is that affirmations can actually change our biology by providing access to the limbic system, the brain's operations center for hope, desire, safety, love, fear, anger, and aggression. The limbic system has connections to the rest of the brain and body, as we have discussed, through hormones and neurotransmitters, in turn affecting all those biological systems proving that thoughts and words are powerful medicine.

Try these affirmations:

- I love and accept myself deeply and completely.
- Each day I become more confident in who I am.
- I have limitless confidence in my abilities.
- I have a natural awareness of all the positive things in my life.

Here is a wonderful resource of <u>free affirmations</u>.

Stress is a part of all of our lives. We have good stress, and unfortunately, we all have bad stress. The purpose of relaxation or meditative exercises is to realize that we do not have to hang onto this stress. We can let it go. We may not be able to change the stressful situations that life presents, but through practice and being in the moment, we can learn to let the physical feelings and physiological consequences of stress pass us by, while we create resilience that can improve the health of our brains.

CHAPTER 13

Eureka!

How to Use Supplements, Herbal Brain Enhancers, and Technology to Prevent Memory Loss and Protect Your Aging Brain

---

"I treat myself pretty good. I take lots of vacations, I eat well, I take supplements, I do mercury detox, I get plenty of sleep, I drink plenty of water, and I stay away from drama and stress."
—Reba McEntire, country music artist

There is a lot of wisdom in Reba's words, and if you have reached this far in the book, and read it from cover to cover, I hope you find her right on point, as I do. I have intentionally left a chapter covering supplements and technology for last, because my message is that *lifestyle is medicine*. Communities of individuals, as famously reported by writer Dan Buettner in his book *The Blue Zones*[65], did not hit the one-hundred year mark with sharp minds and healthy bodies simply because they took pills that made them smarter. The foundation of *The Blue Zones* is a lifestyle that integrates everything we have discussed here. Prevention of memory loss and protection of the aging brain do not come from an anti-inflammatory diet, if sleep is disrupted on a regular basis. They do not come, despite a habit of exercise or commitment to movement, when the body is fueled with processed foods and sugar. They do not come when we fail to take time, on a regular basis, for play, relaxation, and non-judgmental attention to thoughts and sensations, as is the case in a practice of mindfulness. They do not come unless we embrace our spiritual sense of purpose, know who we are and what our job is, for the time we exist in our mortal bodies. Whatever the expression of that purpose, it almost always involves connection to other human beings, one way or another. Just as the functional biological systems are connected and influence one another, so too are the lifestyle factors. Where one pushes, the other pulls. To be sure, this is a juggling act, but those who master the art of juggling know that the most important thing they can do to be successful, besides practice, is relax. Thinking too much about the balls that are in the air inevitably results in one being dropped. It is another form of mindfulness.

With that thought, I will share a few pearls I have learned over the years as a holistic integrative neurologist about supplements, herbs, and — what I find the most exciting — technology. All of the technology I will discuss with you has been cleared by the U.S. Food and Drug Administration. This means that the companies that develop and promote the technology have provided scientific evidence to support the use of their product for its stated purpose. Some of these, I use in my clinical practice today, and others are on the horizon.

When I see patients in my office for my _Brain Tune Up!_ program, they undergo a battery of blood tests during their first visit. These blood tests measure vitamins, minerals, electrolytes, detoxification markers, hormones, inflammatory markers, and levels of antioxidant capacity. Later, if indicated, I may order more advanced testing, such as heavy metal analysis, food sensitivity testing, or a comprehensive analysis of stool, to look at markers of digestion, inflammation, infection, and the health and diversity of the gut microbiome. However, many of my patients can do quite well with the foundational labs only. Why? Because, as my friend and mentor, Dr. Norman Shealy, a pioneer in holistic medicine and a neurosurgeon by training says, "Everything affects everything." Does sleep clear toxins from the brain? The answer should be a resounding "yes," if you recall our discussion of the glymphatic system. Does food choice influence gut inflammation, lead to greater microbial diversity, and improve antioxidant capacity in brain? Heck, yes! Do mindfulness, deep breathing, optimal heart rate variability, and affirmations influence hormones such as cortisol, and thereby dampen its effect on the hippocampus, in turn improving memory, learning, and creativity? You get the picture. However, most of the patients I see in my office are in what I call "crash and burn mode." They are already quite sick, whether it is with Alzheimer's disease, Parkinson's, multiple sclerosis, ALS, or chronic migraines, and for them, especially when deficiencies are identified, some supplementation may be helpful. Since this book is intended as a stand-alone guide, and does not require that you go and have your blood tested, I will tell you what I see commonly, and how you can use this information in your life, without blood tests.

By and large, a framework to think about supplements can be laid out as follows:

1. The use of vitamins and minerals, where the aim is to restore optimal levels of these micronutrients;

2. The use of super-therapeutic doses of vitamins, minerals, or other biochemically active compounds to achieve a pharmacological effect, as measured by a disease state outcome (such as high dose riboflavin to reduce migraine frequency), or a physiological effect (such as the use of L-arginine, an amino acid, to increase nitric oxide levels in tissues — a potent blood vessel dilator). Since the focus of this book is to share the message of lifestyle medicine to protect the brain, I am going to limit my discussion of the use of super-therapeutic doses of vitamins, minerals, or other biochemically active compounds to treat disease states, here.

3. The use of an herbal or botanical supplement for its potential benefit in a manner that cannot be accomplished through food

synergy, because that supplement is either a whole food itself, not otherwise found in food, or not found in food in sufficient quantities to make consuming it in its natural state feasible.

In my office, there are a few supplements that my patients almost always need, based on testing:

1. A high-quality omega 3 fish oil supplement, consisting of at least 1,000 mg of DHA and EPA combined;
2. A probiotic containing a blend of carefully chosen microbes, in concentrations sufficient to have an impact on gut microbial diversity and balance, strengthening the gut-immune barrier, contributing to the production of short chain fatty acids, and improving overall bowel function;
3. Vitamin D, in the form of D3;
4. Zinc;
5. Magnesium; and
6. Folate.

OMEGA 3 FISH OIL

Concentrated fish oil containing a combination of docosahexaenoic acid (DHA) and eicosapentaenoic acid (EPA) provides the form of omega-3 fatty acids found in animals such as cold water fatty fish and grass-fed beef. These molecules are a key component of cell membranes and play a direct and indirect role in resolving inflammation. As with much of what has been discussed in this book, inflammation is neither all "good" or all "bad," and what is really of interest here is the idea of immune balance. Countering the effects of omega-3 fatty acids are the important omega-6 fatty acids, represented by arachidonic acid. So, while not to be undervalued, there is no need to supplement with omega-6 fatty acids. The excessive quantities of these polyunsaturated fatty acids in the American diet is felt to be due largely to the introduction of vegetable oils over the past century. By contrast, an evolutionary perspective on human health suggests that our ancestors had much lower consumption of omega-6 fatty acids, and much higher consumption of omega-3. It would not be unusual to see a patient in my office with an omega-6 to omega-3 ratio of 15:1. Taking into account this hunter-gatherer perspective, the goal, through diet modification and additional supplementation, is to lower that ratio to a range between 2:1 and 5:1. These ratios have been associated with lower rates of recurrent heart attack, reduced rectal cancer proliferation, reduced risk of breast cancer, improved inflammatory control of rheumatoid arthritis, and improvement in asthma control[66]. In the brain, higher intake of omega-3 fatty acids has been linked to a slowing of cognitive decline and a reduction in Alzheimer's pathology. In an animal model of Alzheimer's disease, relatively long-term omega-3 fatty acid supplementation (at least 10% of the total lifespan) improved measures of learning and memory, while reducing the amount of amyloid beta-42 in the brain and limiting the amount of neuronal loss[67]. DHA, in particular, appears to promote the connections between nerve cells (synaptogenesis).

The processing of fish to extract these oils has come under scrutiny. For example, one report of fish oil supplements in New Zealand found the samples to be highly oxidized and they did not meet label content of omega-3 fatty acids[68]. In my office, I recommend only pharmaceutical-grade fish oil supplements in the natural triglyceride form, to provide optimal digestion and absorption. Dose recommended: 1,000 mg of combined DHA and EPA daily.

PROBIOTICS

Probiotics that include *Lactobacillus* and *Bifidobacterium* species have been found to confer a wide variety of benefits to gastrointestinal health. Given the gut-brain connection, a healthy gut is the foundation of a healthy brain. The blend of probiotics used in my office has been shown to improve the absorption of minerals, protect the gut lining from harmful bacteria, support gut-associated immune tissue (responsible for the first line of defense against inflammatory and infectious threats), reduce intestinal permeability, and improve overall microbial balance. Look for a combination of *Lactobacillus acidophilus, Lactobacillus paracasei, Lactobacillus plantarum, Lactobacillus rhamnosus, Bifidobacterium lactis, Bifidobacterium bifidum* (20 billion Colony Forming Units collectively, and *Saccharomyces boulardii,* 2 billion CFU). Here is an excellent, but technical, review of the <u>mechanisms of action of probiotics</u>.

VITAMIN D

Vitamin D is a fat-soluble vitamin that serves numerous functions. While most people know about vitamin D and its role in bone formation, the focus here is its role in the brain. The main source of vitamin D is ultraviolet light from the sun, while about 20% comes from diet. However, sunlight exposure in modern life is significantly less than that of our ancestors, on average, and when we do go out in the sun, we wear a lot of sun-protective clothing and slather our skin in chemical-laden sunblock. After all, the message has been to protect the skin from direct sun exposure. Furthermore, our food supply and food consumption habits, with a trend toward a higher carbohydrate and lower fat diet, likely contributes to the commonly observed suboptimal levels, when measured. Some drugs also increase the breakdown of vitamin D in the body. A paper published in the journal *Nutrition Research* in 2011 found an overall prevalence of vitamin D deficiency in the U.S. of 41% (as measured by the *National Health and Nutrition Examination Survey 2005 to 2006*). These researchers defined deficiency as a level of 20 ng/ml or less. When examined this way, vitamin D deficiency was significantly more common among those who had no college education, those who were obese, individuals with overall poor health status, those who had hypertension, low "good cholesterol" (HDL), or who did not consume dairy[69]. In my office, I want my patients to have vitamin D levels in the range of 60-100 ng/ml. If you consider how common vitamin D deficiency is, when defined by a level of 20 or less, you can imagine that the percent who present with a level in the optimal range for the brain is virtually nil. Remember, those in my office are already affected by neurological disease. Low levels of vitamin D have been associated with the risk of all causes of dementia, including Alzheimer's disease, and with multiple sclerosis. In the brain, vitamin D acts as a steroid hormone, particularly in areas related to learning and memory. Vitamin D regulates nerve growth factor production, neurotransmitter release, calcium balance, oxidative stress mechanisms, and the immune system's inflammatory responses[70]. In the Alzheimer's brain, it appears that vitamin D may help to decrease the burden of amyloid beta-42, and levels in the range of 60 ng/mL for people who have MS result in less disease activity and less disability progression[71]. Dose recommended: 5,000 IU in the form of Vitamin D3.

ZINC

The worldwide prevalence of zinc deficiency is significant. Deficiency from zinc malnutrition was estimated in a 2002 report by the World Health Organization to be associated with 1.8 million deaths annually[72]. Estimates of the percent of the population at risk for inadequate zinc intake varies greatly from 12% to 66%, depending on the methods used[73]. Nevertheless, the problem remains substantial and when it comes to the aging brain, evidence suggests that low zinc intake among older adults is a serious problem. Calculations for adults 60 years and older from the third National Health and Nutrition Examination Survey (1988-1994) found that inadequate intake of zinc ranged from

35% to 45% of men and women[74]. Zinc has a number of roles to play throughout the body, including its support for enzyme activity, immune function, protein synthesis, wound healing, cell division, growth and development. In the brain, the highest levels of zinc are found in the hippocampus and in the retina of the eye (which can be thought of as an extension of the brain). Disturbances in brain zinc can occur either because of deficient intake or absorption, decreased utilization by the body, or increased loss through the colon, and this results in problems with learning, memory, mood, and behavior. In Alzheimer's disease, the precise role of zinc remains controversial. Zinc itself has been associated with the processing of the amyloid precursor protein into amyloid beta-42 peptides, and the accumulation of the amyloid plaques in the brain. However, this appears to be less a problem of zinc excess as it does the balance of how the body utilizes zinc in the face of excess copper, and the role that zinc plays as part of the brain's response to inflammatory signals from the environment[75]. In my office, serum zinc and copper levels are routinely measured, and I look for a level between 90 – 110 mcg/dL, with copper approximately the same. It is quite common to find low levels of serum zinc and high levels of serum copper. The addition of zinc as a supplement will not only help maintain good levels of zinc, but it will help to reduce excess copper. I recommend supplementation with a zinc chelate for optimal absorption, such has zinc picolinate or zinc bisglycinate, in a dose range of 30 – 50 mg daily.

MAGNESIUM

Magnesium, like zinc, is an element which is essential to numerous biochemical reactions throughout the body. It serves functions such as the contraction and relaxation of muscle, the formation of bone, and the maintenance of blood sugar balance. It plays an important part in ATP metabolism, and is therefore critical to the health of mitochondria.

In the brain, magnesium helps to control the activation of NMDA receptors, specialized proteins found on the surface of neurons activated by the excitatory neurotransmitter glutamate. While glutamate-related pathways are important for learning and memory, excessive glutamate activity is thought to be toxic to brain cells and to lead to neurodegeneration[76]. Low magnesium has been associated with type 2 diabetes, high blood pressure, atherosclerotic disease, sudden cardiac death, osteoporosis, asthma, migraines, seizures, and colon cancer. A 2012 paper by Andrea Rosanoff, PhD suggests that nearly half the U.S. population consumes less than the required amount of magnesium from food.[77] Aside from poor intake, causes of low magnesium include alcohol use, intestinal dysfunction (such as diarrhea, Inflammatory Bowel Syndrome and Celiac disease), medication, and stress. Among the medications that can interfere with magnesium absorption are the Proton Pump Inhibitors (PPIs), prescribed and over-the-counter, to block the production of acid in the stomach. Long-term use of PPIs, because they disrupt an essential biological function of the digestive system, have been associated with a number of adverse health outcomes, including hip fractures, pneumonia, C. *difficile* intestinal infections (which can be fatal), kidney disease, and even the risk of dementia, including Alzheimer's[78,79].

Measurement of intracellular tissue magnesium can be accomplished most accurately with an ExaTest® (IntraCellular Diagnostics, Inc.). But a more cost-effective compromise is a red blood cell magnesium (RBC Magnesium). I look for an RBC Magnesium of 5.2 – 6.4 mg/dL. Critical to the use of magnesium as a food supplement is its absorbability in the oral form. Common, over-the-counter magnesium preparations are magnesium carbonate and magnesium oxide. Unfortunately, they are not readily bioavailable, and can lead to gastrointestinal distress. Instead, I recommend a chelated oral form of magnesium. Here, elemental magnesium is bound to amino acids such as glycine, lysine, or the dicarboxylic acid malate to form a salt, in a dose of approximately 400 mg per day. Dr. Norman Shealy has suggested that transdermal absorption of magnesium may be superior to oral absorption[80]. Topical magnesium preparations are readily available through commercial vendors.

FOLATE

Folate is a member of the B-vitamin family and is sometimes referred to as B9. I have debated about my recommendations on folate supplementation, and I will explain. There are certain instances where empiric folate supplementation is absolutely appropriate. Periconceptual folate supplementation reduces the risk of having children born with neural tube defects and autism. This is why standard prenatal vitamins contain folate. Furthermore, there is a long list of folate-depleting drugs, and if it is absolutely necessary to take one of those medications, consideration should be given to supplementation with folate. The biochemistry of folate involves the support of pathways in the body that affect synthesis of neurotransmitters like dopamine, norepinephrine, and serotonin, estrogen metabolism, the manufacture of glutathione, and the behavior of our DNA. Pretty important when it comes to the brain! Much of this happens through complex chemistry involving the transfer of a single carbon molecule, called a methyl group ($-CH_3$), made possible by folate in its active form, L-5-methyltetrahydrofolate.

The "methylation" of DNA acts as an off-switch. It suppresses the transcription, or reading and decoding, of that portion of the DNA. This is epigenetics, the way to alter the expression of our genes without changing the genes themselves. No doubt, our cells normally execute epigenetic commands on a regular basis as part of homeostatic control. The question arises whether "forcing" these pathways through administration of high dose folate might have adverse consequences. If, for example, a gene that suppresses cancer (called a "tumor suppressor gene") is turned off through methylation, then the consequence could be an increased risk of cancer. As one example reported in the *Annals of Internal Medicine*, the methylation (resulting in inactivation) of a normal gene involved in the repair of damaged DNA, called BRCA1, results in an increased risk of ovarian cancer[81]. Folate as a therapeutic modality is complex, as you can see. In the clinic setting, besides measuring serum folate, it is possible to evaluate methylation biochemistry a number of different ways through laboratory testing. In the absence of a functional medicine practitioner familiar with the use of these tests, it may be difficult to know how much folate to take as a food supplement, and as I have suggested, more is not necessarily better.

As the availability of folate diminishes, levels of an amino acid called homocysteine may go up. It turns out that elevated blood homocysteine levels and low folate levels are independent predictors of the development of dementia, including Alzheimer's disease[82]. In my clinic, I test homocysteine and other related measures, and I replace with supplemental folate where indicated. What can you do if you are reading this book? In short, you can eat green, leafy vegetables. Research from Rush University in Chicago and Tufts University in Boston reported in the journal *Neurology* that consumption of as little as 1 serving per day of green leafy vegetables — rich in folate and a number of phytonutrients (phylloquinone, lutein, kaempferol), nitrate, alpha-tocopherol (vitamin E) — was associated with slower cognitive decline among 960 participants of the Memory and Aging Project, ages 58-99 years[83].

HERBAL SUPPLEMENTS AS BRAIN ENHANCERS

There are a few remarkable compounds that fall under the category of herbal or botanical supplements. They show potential benefit, either as a whole food, a compound not otherwise found in food, or not found in food in sufficient quantities to make consuming them in their natural state feasible. The root herb turmeric, an ingredient used in curry, has been implicated as the reason for the lower prevalence of Alzheimer's disease in India. The key constituent of turmeric is the family of phenols known as curcuminoids, which have potent antioxidant and anti-inflammatory properties. I encourage my patients to use turmeric liberally in their cooking or added to a smoothie. As a supplement, the turmeric extract, Curcuma longa, is available and generally combined with bioperine (a black pepper extract) or bound molecularly to phosphatidylcholine to make the curcumin more readily absorbable. The recommended dose of curcumin as a supplement is 500 mg daily.

Resveratrol, another phenol, is naturally found in grape skins and berries, and in minute quantities in red wine. Like turmeric and its curcuminoids, resveratrol may exert its effect through antioxidant and anti-inflammatory mechanisms. In a randomized, double-blind, placebo-controlled trial, resveratrol 500 mg orally once daily, escalating to a dose of 1,000 mg twice daily had the effect of stabilizing spinal fluid and blood levels of a biomarker that normally declines in Alzheimer's disease. It should be noted that the dose of resveratrol used in the study was quite large, and it was associated with adverse side effects, such as nausea, diarrhea, and weight loss.[84] It would not be possible to drink enough red wine to get sufficient quantities of resveratrol. I recommend resveratrol in the "trans-" form, a configuration with more biological activity, at a dose of 100 mg daily.

The root from the plant *Withania somnifera*, called ashwagandha, used in Ayurvedic medicine, may have the effect of reducing amyloid plaque pathology in the brain by enhancing clearance of amyloid beta-42. However, while this has been studied in a mouse model of Alzheimer's disease[85] the benefit in human beings is unknown. In addition to its impact on Alzheimer's plaques, ashwagandha is used as an adrenal adaptogen to temper the effects of cortisol, our stress hormone, on the body. I find the easiest way to benefit from ashwagandha is to purchase the ground up organic root powder and use approximately 1 gram (¼ to ½ tsp., depending on the concentration) in a smoothie.

Lion's mane mushroom or Hericium erinaceus (also called yamabushitake by the Japanese) has been used to boost the production of nerve growth factor in the brain, and in doing so, stimulate synaptic connections between nerve cells[86]. As with ashwagandha, the benefit of Lion's mane mushroom has been studied in a mouse model of Alzheimer's disease, and demonstrated benefit[87], although the advantage to human beings with the disease or used preventatively remains undetermined. Lion's mane is a food, and while it can be taken in encapsulated form, it can also be enjoyed as a key ingredient in recipes prepared in your kitchen. It is also available in powdered form, where a serving of approximately 2 grams can be mixed into a smoothie or added to a hot cup of coffee.

TECHNOLOGY TO PROTECT AND ENHANCE THE BRAIN

Many years ago, I discovered I had a fondness for technology. I grew up in the days of analog stereo systems. (I still have a good collection of vinyl LPs.) I knew McIntosh as a state-of-the-art tube amplifier before the name was borrowed (and the "a" added) by Steve Jobs for what is now an icon of the late 20th and early 21st century. From designing imaginary starships on giant pieces of graph paper as a teenager, I graduated to building my own computers when the fastest connection to the Internet involved a dial-up modem. In 2001, before the idea of functional medicine ever occurred to me, I was approached by a biotechnology company representative to see if I might be interested in learning more about vagus nerve stimulation for treatment of epileptic seizures. At the time, her company was called Cyberonics (now LivaNova), and they had developed a device, Food and Drug Administration-approved since 1997, to help people whose seizures could not be controlled on medication alone. Eight years later, in 2005, the company received approval for treatment of severe, recurrent depression.

The device is pretty straightforward. There is a part called a "pulse generator," a disk-shaped piece of metal that contains what I would describe as a small computer, fit with a long-life battery. It is thin, and about two to three inches in diameter. It must be implanted by a surgeon who, with the patient under general anesthesia, creates a pocket under the skin on the chest, adjacent to the left armpit. A second incision is made in the mid-to-lower portion of the neck on the left side, where the left vagus nerve is identified alongside the common carotid artery. This part of the vagus nerve is transmitting nerve signals primarily toward the brain, rather than away from it. (You may recall that the descending vagus nerve sends signals to the vocal cords, heart, lungs, and digestive system.) A lead wire is wrapped around the left vagus nerve, and tunneled under the skin, where it is connected to the pulse generator. The patient is sutured at the incision sites on the neck and chest, anesthesia is stopped, and the operation is over. During the coming months, the pulse generator is programmed to deliver a small current of electricity to the vagus nerve, and thereby stimulate higher brain centers to help control seizures and elevate mood.

It is thought that the VNS® has multiple mechanisms to account for its efficacy[88,89,90,91]. These include:

- increasing concentrations of neurotransmitters, such as norepinephrine, in key areas of the brain, including the amygdala, hippocampus, and prefrontal cortex;
- increasing serotonin activity through a structure known as the dorsal raphe nucleus;
- positive effects on the inhibitory neurotransmitter GABA or its receptors;
- a positive effect on immune system activity in the brain — bearing in mind that the hippocampus, a structure often involved in seizures, has many cortisol receptors;
- positive effects on neuroplasticity (how nerve cells wire together); and,

- changes in regional brain blood flow and glucose metabolism.

While VNS® technology is not frequently discussed in holistic medicine circles, I would argue that its efficacy is entirely in line with holistic principles, all the way down to its effect as a modulator of inflammation and limbic system activity. My point is also that the most optimal scenario for applying the principles of VNS® technology is in the context of addressing cellular health in the brain and the body. This comes back full circle to the modifiable lifestyle factors and their effect on each of the functional biological systems. There are a lot of "gadget gurus" in the world of holistic medicine, and they may truly have something to offer, but it is not possible to expect a long term, sustained outcome, without addressing the foundation first. In my personal experience, I see individuals who have dialed in their nutrition, but are either not exercising, not sleeping, or not practicing stress resilience. It should come as no surprise that the incomplete approach does not result in satisfactory improvement. These shortcomings cannot be compensated for by the use of technology.

Energy is a powerful tool, when it comes to healing and protecting the brain. We have already discussed the role that sunlight plays in brain health, in the chapter on sleep. Another earthly interest in energy medicine is the subject of earthing or grounding. The premise of grounding is the transfer of electrons between the earth and our bodies. Free radicals (or oxidants) were discussed in the sections on oxidative stress and mitochondria. With grounding, a walk on grass, dirt, or sand (like the beach) allows for the flow of electrons into the body to help mitigate excess free radical damage, reduce inflammation, and balance hormones. A good review on this subject and the potential health implications can be found here. While there is technology available to enhance your experience of this interesting phenomenon, I suggest simply taking off your shoes and going outside.

Just as sunlight and earth are healing forces, technology can harness aspects of nature to provide healing benefit to the brain. The idea is that light in the red or near-infrared range protects tissue that has either been injured, is degenerating, or is at risk for dying. Using light-emitting diodes that flicker at a specific rate (40 Hz), it may be possible to reduce the burden of amyloid beta-42 in the Alzheimer's brain and alter the behavior of the microglia[92]. In a study published by Massachusetts Institute of Technology researchers, there was a 40-50% reduction in amyloid beta-42 protein in the hippocampi of mice, in an experimental model of Alzheimer's disease. The flicker rate of the LEDs mimics a brain wave frequency known as gamma oscillations, normally present during activities involving learning and memory. This technology has moved out of the laboratory and into human trials. A study of photobiomodulation (PBM) is underway to improve brain function in dementia[93]. The basis for the research was a case report of 5 patients with mild to moderately severe dementia who were treated with a PBM device. The study subjects experienced improvements on standard cognitive testing, such as the Mini Mental Status Examination, after 12 weeks of therapy[94]. For those who cannot wait for the results of the clinical trial, photobiomodulation devices can be purchased for personal use. While not FDA-approved in the United States for Alzheimer's disease, they may still be acquired under guidelines that define them as low-risk general wellness devices. The company is called Vielight, and the device under study in the current clinical trial is the <u>Vielight Neuro Gamma</u>®. They are TUV-certified[95] as safe for consumer use.

Sound can also have a therapeutic effect. Here, the concept is called binaural beats, and it was popularized by a biophysicist named Gerald Oster[96]. In this case, sounds delivered separately to each ear elicit specific responses in the brain. Brain wave frequencies associated with different states of consciousness, such as relaxation, meditation, creativity, focus, concentration, alertness, or sleep can be provoked by these recordings. Many binaural beats are available for purchase or for free. Make sure you enjoy them with headphones, to achieve the proper result.

Two other areas of technology that impact brain function are transcranial electrical and magnetic stimulation. These devices exert their effect noninvasively, through placement on or near the scalp, and send their energy to the brain. Broadly, these are called neurostimulation devices, although one could argue that *all* the devices I have presented are neurostimulators, which I think makes an important point about neuroplasticity, in general. In order for neuroplasticity to take place, the brain needs a reason to change. This reason is like a set of commands, instructions that tell the brain what you want it to do. It can come through exercise and intentional movement. It can come through spiritual affirmations and other self-talk. It can come through hormones, neurotransmitters, and cytokines, all of which are influenced by food, sleep, and human connection.

Transcranial electrical stimulation is broadly divided into Cranial Electrotherapy Stimulation (CES, for short, a form of Alternating Current Stimulation) and Transcranial Direct Current Stimulation (tDCS). With transcranial electrical stimulation, a low level of electrical current is delivered to targeted areas of the brain to achieve specific results. The effect is achieved through two processes called Long-term potentiation (LTP) and Long-term depression (LTD).

There is an old expression in neuroscience attributed to Donald Hebb, a Canadian psychologist, which goes like this: *Neurons that fire together wire together.* Put in another way, nerve pathways that are frequently activated tend to be reinforced in the brain; the opposite is also true: the nerve pathways which are not frequently activated tend to be weak.

Let's use a concrete example. Do you play a musical instrument? On your first lesson, you may learn the basic fingering of a few chords on the guitar, but it feels awkward. Practice for 30 minutes every day for two weeks, and the chords will come much more naturally. This is neuroplasticity, and this is neurons that are wiring together after repeatedly firing together. Now, maybe you played guitar (as I did) in high school and college. Thirty years later, you may pick up that instrument and vaguely remember the chords, but you are rusty, and the nerve pathways do not fire as well. What if you were new to the guitar and you used an electrical device on your scalp that "primed" the connections between key nerve cells in your brain involved in playing guitar. It did not make you automatically know how to play those chords, but perhaps instead of becoming more comfortable with them in two weeks, you were able to learn them in only one week. Here is the textbook definition: LTP is a form of activity-dependent plasticity which results in persistent enhancement of synaptic transmission. LTD is an example in which the efficacy of synaptic transmission is reduced[97]. Both are important if you want to change a previously hardwired behavior.

It appears that these electrical devices do not actually cause the nerve cells to fire, but they alter their threshold for firing, or their "excitability." This amplifies the effects that you are trying to achieve (to potentiate or suppress the pathway). Research into the physiology of transcranial direct current stimulation suggest that it has effects on non-neuronal structures as well, such as glia and the endothelial cells that line the blood-brain barrier through a process called "electro-permeation[98]." I can imagine the role this technology might one day play in treatment of "Leaky Brain Syndrome"! One difference between the direct current and alternating current stimulation is that the latter can more easily manipulate the normal up-and-down oscillations of brain waves, a process called "entrainment," because of the nature of alternating current.

Reminiscent of the effect of binaural beats, oscillatory activity plays a central role in regulating thinking and memory, mood, cerebral blood flow, and neurotransmitter levels[99]. One study of transcranial direct current stimulation looked at the effect of polarity changes on GABA and glutamate. When subjects were stimulated using the positive terminal (the anode), the result was locally reduced GABA (suggesting this has an excitatory effect), whereas when subjects were stimulated using the negative terminal (the cathode), the result was reduced glutaminergic activity (suggesting this has an inhibitory effect)[100]. Remember that GABA is an inhibitory neurotransmitter, whereas glutamate is an excitatory neurotransmitter.

In a separate paper using a Cranial Electrotherapy Stimulator, the researchers noted an increase in spinal fluid levels of serotonin, beta-endorphin, GABA, and DHEA, together with decreased levels of cortisol and tryptophan[101]. Returning briefly to our discussion of photobiomodulation earlier in this chapter, it has been found that the brains of patients with Alzheimer's disease have disrupted brain signaling, specifically, alterations in gamma rhythm, an oscillatory frequency in the range of 31 to 140 cycles per second. Recall that the therapeutic effect of the flickering light occurred at 40 cycles per second, the upshot of which is to restore the normal gamma rhythm of the brain. So, it appears that sound, light, and electricity all have overlapping impacts.

One other modality that is not discussed here in detail is repetitive Transcranial Magnetic Stimulation (rTMS). This FDA-approved technology is used primarily by psychiatrists and psychologists as a tool for office-based treatment of depression, bipolar disorder, Post-Traumatic Stress Disorder, Obsessive Compulsive Disorder, and adult Attention Deficit Disorder. The combination of cost, technological complexity, and large footprint means it does not lend itself to personal use, and therefore is outside of the goals of this book. However, the concept is similar, and my review of the literature revealed a recently published study in which, perhaps not surprisingly, rTMS was used to reverse amyloid beta-42-induced dysfunction in gamma frequency oscillation associated with working memory[102]. Bear in mind, however, that this was a laboratory study using adult Sprague Dawley rats.

Although transcranial direct current stimulation is limited to research at the present time, tACS or Cranial Electrotherapy Stimulation devices are commercially available and relatively inexpensive. I use two brands of devices in my office and encourage my patients who find them beneficial to purchase one of their own. The Fisher Wallace Stimulator® is FDA-cleared to treat depression, anxiety, and chronic pain. In addition, published research also supports its potential benefit to enhance attention and concentration[103], stress-related cognitive dysfunction[104], and attention-deficit hyperactivity disorder in children and adults[105]. Similar products are sold by Alpha-Stim®, called the Alpha-Stim M® and Alpha-Stim AID®.

Not all Cranial Electrotherapy Stimulation is focused on cognitive functioning. A company called Halo Neuroscience, headed by Stanford-trained MD and neuroscientist Daniel Chao and his co-founder Brett Wingeier, PhD, a biomedical engineer, have developed the Halo Sport®. While currently being marketed for enhancement of motor function in athletes — recall our discussion of long-term potentiation and nerve cell firing thresholds — the Halo Sport® holds promise for those suffering from Parkinson's disease and other movement disorders by facilitating the activation of pathways under conscious control. Here, 20 minutes of use prior to exercise enhances motor pathways and allows for stronger synaptic connections when stimulation is followed by the movement behavior the athlete wishes to reinforce. It reminds me of the old joke sometimes attributed to comedian Jack Benny: "How do you get to Carnegie Hall (the pedestrian asks the taxi driver)?" Answer: "Practice, my man, practice."

Here is the theme: functional medicine is medicine of action. Your provider, whether he is a physician or another practitioner or coach, is merely your guide on this journey, your Obi-Wan Kenobi. But it is you who must ultimately face the challenges and discover the treasure hidden in your innermost cave.

EPILOGUE

The Road Back

Congratulations! You have completed your journey in *The Healthy Brain Toolbox*, and now it is time to enjoy the rewards. The challenges of the road back are two-fold. If you have already taken action, it will be up to you to maintain the enormous benefit you have experienced through the changes and lifestyle strategies recommended in this book. The scientific concepts in **Part 1** have provided you with the vocabulary and knowledge to further your understanding of functional medicine, as it relates to brain health or any other area of health that might interest you. The action steps of **Part 2** have given you the framework for a lifelong plan to prevent memory loss and protect your aging brain.

In my experience, sometimes feeling better (or looking better) in the short run is not enough to sustain momentum, in the long run. It will be important to explore your sense of self-reward — the things that fuel your enthusiasm — to give yourself the needed boost from time-to-time, to prevent unhealthy behaviors from creeping in. Barriers, detours, or diversionary temptations will need to be addressed. For example, as discussed in Chapter 11, you may need to remove inflammatory foods from your cupboard and refrigerator, and either give them away, or donate them. If you have a weekly night out with friends for indulgences and libations, you may need to make it clear to them that this is your new lifestyle, and food options must be available that support your needs. Limit your alcohol. You may even need to seek out new social circles and "hang outs" that back up and reinforce the habits you want to maintain. Use your affirmations on a daily basis to remain clear about who you are and what you want. It is not required that affirmation work take place during sedentary times. Affirmations can be combined with exercise, a perfect occasion to visualize and manifest your goals. Get your sleep. Because sleep is a time for repair, recovery, and reinvigoration, and all the biological processes dependent on sleep discussed in Chapter 9. Take the supplements I have recommended in Chapter 13.

There is still one more discovery to make. In Chapter 2 of this book, I mentioned how social isolation is a major health problem for older adults, and how loneliness is linked to the risk of Alzheimer's disease. The last modifiable risk factor we have to discuss is Connection. As human beings — at the most primitive level — family, friendships, and community are part of who we are and what we do. Certainly, being connected helps to fulfill the other basic needs. We are more likely to find food, water, safety, and shelter, and — obviously — reproduce, if we have the company of other people we know and trust. This has ensured our species success through the millennia. Matthew Lieberman, PhD, director of UCLA's Social Cognitive Neuroscience Lab suggests that social pain — the pain experienced from loss or rejection — is just as powerful as physical pain when we consider its effect on the brain. Lieberman demonstrated his findings using technology called functional MRI. In fact, says Lieberman, "The same brain regions that register the distress of physical pain are also active in situations when we experience social pain," such as rejection or exclusion. "Social pain may not be pleasant in the moment," he continues, "but we would be lost without it." We benefit from acute social pain, like the signal of acute physical pain. It is a call to action. But just as other imbalances within the functional biological systems (Chapter 5) drive inflammation and oxidative stress (Chapter 4), so too does social isolation, when it is persistent[106,107]. It has all the same effects on the brain and the body. Conversely, social connection brings balance to the system, and, according to Lieberman, "is one of the best predictors of happiness and well-being." For more information about Dr. Lieberman's work, watch his 2013 TEDx St. Louis Talk, or explore his book entitled, *Social: Why Our Brains are Wired to Connect* (Crown, 2013).

Not only does the brain function more optimally when we connect to one another, but we are rewarded for doing so. Oxytocin, a hormone produced in the hypothalamus and secreted by the pituitary gland, plays a critical role in love, bonding, positive trusting relationships, maternal care, and sexual behavior, while reducing anxiety and depression. Not surprisingly, then, it turns out that oxytocin has anti-inflammatory effects on the brain[108]. More than likely, it also has antioxidant effects, as demonstrated in the heart[109].

It is no ordinary world that you return to after this journey. You will see it through an entirely new lens called functional medicine. I could have remained a conventional neurologist, prescribing medication for chronic diseases of the nervous system, referring to surgeons to cut out the problem, or succumbing to the default answer — "I don't know" — when my patient asks me, "Why did I get sick?" (The medical terminology is "idiopathic," meaning spontaneous onset of unknown cause.) Like the character Neo in *The Matrix*, I chose to take the "red pill," and my career and way of thinking as a neurologist — my life — was transformed forever. For me, that came on one of the rainiest days in the recorded history of Scottsdale, Arizona, a city in the desert. The question of whether this information has changed you, of course, is for you to decide.

END NOTES

Chapter 1

1 Deokar AJ, Bouldin ED, Edwards VJ. Increased confusion and memory loss in households, 20-11 Behavioral Risk Factor Surveillance System. *Prev Chronic Dis* 2015;140430

2 https://www.nationalmssociety.org/About-the-Society/News/Preliminary-Results-of-MS-Prevalence-Study

3 http://migraineresearchfoundation.org/about-migraine/migraine-facts/

Chapter 2

4 Rodriguez-Vietez E, Saint-Aubert L, Carter SF, et al. Diverging longitudinal changes in astrocytosis and amyloid PET in autosomal dominant Alzheimer's disease. *Brain* 2016;139(3):922-936.

5 Kac G, Perez-Escamilla RP. Nutrition transition and obesity prevention through the life course. *International Journal of Obesity* 2013;Supplement 3:S6-S8.

6 Nwankwo T, Yoon SS, Gu Q. Hypertension among adults in the United States: National Health and Nutrition Examination Survey, 2011-2012. *NCHS Data Brief* 2013;Oct(133):1-8.

7 https://www.cdc.gov/media/releases/2017/p0718-diabetes-report.html

8 https://aasm.org/rising-prevalence-of-sleep-apnea-in-u-s-threatens-public-health/

9 https://www.apa.org/news/press/releases/stress/2011/final-2011.pdf

10 https://assets.americashealthrankings.org/app/uploads/2017annualreport.pdf

11 Nicholson NR. A review of social isolation: an important but under-addressed condition in older adults. *J Prim Prev* 2012;33(2-3)137-152.

Chapter 3

12 Benjamin EJ, Blaha MJ, Chiuve SE, et al. on behalf of the American Heart Association Statistics Committee and Stroke Statistics Subcommittee. Heart disease and stroke statistics—2017 update: a report from the American Heart Association. *Circulation.* 2017;135:e229-e445.

13 http://www.thennt.com/nnt/anti-hypertensives-to-prevent-death-heart-attacks-and-strokes/

14 http://www.cochrane.org/CD006742/HTN_benefits-of-antihypertensive-drugs-for-mild-hypertension -are-unclear

Chapter 5

15 Vogt NM, Kerby RL, Dill-McFarland KA, et al. Gut microbiome alterations in Alzheimer's disease. *Scientific Reports.* October 2017;7:e13537.

16 Cekanaviciute E, Yoo BB, Runia TF et al. Gut bacteria from multiple sclerosis patients modulate human T-cells and exacerbate symptoms in mouse models. *PNAS* October 3, 2017;114(40):10713-10718.

17 Wu S, Yi J, Zhang Y-g, et al. Leaky intestine and impaired microbiome in an amyotrophic lateral sclerosis mouse model. *Physiological Reports* April 2015;3(4):e12356.

18 Perez-Parko P, Hartog M, Garssen J et al. Microbes tickling your tummy: the importance of the gut-brain axis in Parkinson's disease. *Curr Behav Neurosci Rep* 2017;4(4):361-368.

19 Dos Santos EF, Busanello ENB, Migllioranza A. Evidence that folic acid deficiency is a major determinant of hyperhomocysteinemia in Parkinson's disease. *Metab Brain Dis* 2009;24(2):257-259.

20 Samson TR, Debelius JW, Thron T, et al. Gut microbiota regulate motor deficits and neuroinflammation in a model of Parkinson's disease. *Cell* 2016;167(6):1469-1480.

21 Groschwitz KR, Hogan SP. Intestinal barrier function: molecular regulation and disease pathogenesis. *J of Allergy and Clinical Immunology* 2009;124(1):3-22.

22 Fasano A. Zonulin, regulation of tight junctions, and autoimmune disease. *Annals of the New York Academy of Science* 2012;1258(1):25-33.

23   Mawanda F, Wallace R. Can infections cause Alzheimer's disease? *Epidemiologic Reviews* 2013;35:161-180.

24   Pawate S, Sriram S. The role of infections in the pathogenesis and course of multiple sclerosis. *Annals of Indian Academy of Neurology* 2010;13(2):80-86.

25   Correale J, Farez M, Razzitte G. Helminth Infections associated with multiple sclerosis induce regulatory B-cells. *Annals of Neurology* 2008;64(2):187-199.

26   Lee JW, Lee YK, Yuk DY, et al. Neuro-inflammation induced by lipopolysaccharide causes cognitive impairment through enhancement of beta-amyloid generation. *Journal of Neuroinflammation* 2008;5:37.

27   Escribano BM, Medina-Fernandez FJ, Agular-Lugue M, et al. Lipopolysaccharide binding protein and oxidative stress in a multiple sclerosis model. *Neurotherapeutics* 2017;14(1):199-211

28   Liu M, Bing G. Lipopolysaccharide animal models for Parkinson's disease. *Parkinson's disease* 2011; Article ID 327089.

29   Zhang R, Miller RG, Gascon R, et al. Circulating endotoxin and systemic immune activation in sporadic amyotrophic lateral sclerosis (sALS). J *Neuroimmunology* 2009;206(102):121-124.

30   Tistra JS, Clauson CL, Niedernhofer LJ, Robbins PD. NF-kB in aging and disease. *Aging and Disease* 2011;2(6):449-465.

31   Sullan MJ, Asken BM, Jaffee MS, et al. Glymphatic system disruption as a mediator of brain trauma and chronic traumatic encephalopathy. *Neurosci Biobehav Rev* 2018;84:316-324.

32   Kress BT, Liff JJ, Xia M, et al. Impairment of paravascular clearance pathways in the aging brain. *Annals of Neurology* 2014;76(8):845-61.

33   Trasoff-Conway JM, Carare RO, Osorio RS, et al. Clearance systems in the brain-implications for Alzheimer's disease. Nat Rev Neurol 2015;11(8):457-470.

34   (+)-7R,8S-dihyrodiol-9S,10R-epoxy-benzo[a]pyrene

35   Yoon E, Barbar A, Choudhary M, Kutner M. Acetaminophen-induced hepatotoxicity: a comprehensive update. *J Clin Transl Hepatol* 2016;4(2):131-142.

36   Genuis SJ, Kelln KL. Toxicant exposure and bioaccumulation: a common and potentially reversible cause of cognitive dysfunction and dementia. *Behavioral Neurology* 2015;Article ID:620143.

37   Empting LD. Neurological and neuropsychiatric syndrome features of mold and mycotoxin exposure. *Toxicol Ind Health* 2009 Oct-Nov;25(9-10):577-81.

38   Langston JW. The MPTP story. J Parkinsons Dis 2017;7(Suppl 1):S11-S22.

39 Tanriverdi F, Karaca Z, Unluhizarci K, Kelestimur F. *Stress* 2007;10(1):13-25.

40 Zandi PP, Carlson MC, Plassman BL, Welsh-Bohmer KA, Mayer LS, Steffens DC, et al. Hormone replacement therapy and incidence of Alzheimer disease in older women: the Cache County Study. *JAMA.* 2002;;288(17):2123–2129.

41 Rivera CM, Grossardt BR, Rhodes DJ, et al. Increased mortality for neurological and mental diseases following early bilateral oophorectomy. *Neuroepidemiology* 2009;33:32-40.

42 Rocca, WA, Grossardt BR, Shuster LT. Oophorectomy, menopause, estrogen treatment, and cognitive aging: clinical evidence for a window of opportunity. *Brain Res* 2011;1379:188-198.

43 Chong JY, Rowland LP, Utiger RD. Hashimoto's encephalopathy: syndrome or myth? *Arch Neurol* 2003;60(2):164-171.

44 Bioemer J, Bhattacharya S, Amin R, Suppiramaniam V. Impaired insulin signaling and mechanisms of memory loss. *Prog Mol Biol Transl Sci* 2014;121:413-419.

Chapter 6

45 Micha R, Penalvo JL, Cudhea F, et al. Association between dietary factors and mortality from heart disease, stroke, and type 2 diabetes in the United States. *JAMA* 2017;317(9):912-924.

Chapter 7

46 Corder EH, Saunders AM, Strittmatter WJ, et al. Gene dose of apolipoprotein type 4 allele and the risk of Alzheimer's disease in late-onset families. *Science* 1993;261:921-923.

Chapter 8

47 Cerebral Autosomal Dominant Arteriopathy with Subcortical Infarcts and Leukoencephalopathy. For more information, see https://rarediseases.org/rare-diseases/cadasil/

Chapter 9

48 Oliveira de Almeida CM, Malheiro A. Sleep, immunity, and shift workers: a review. *Sleep Sci* 2016;9(3):164-168.

49   Poroyko VA, Carerras A, Khalyfa A, et al. Chronic sleep disruption alters gut microbiota, induces systemic and adipose tissue inflammation, and insulin resistance in mice. *Scientific Reports* 2016; Article 35405.

50   Benedict C, Vogel H, Jonas W, et al. Gut microbiota and glucometabolic alterations to recurrent partial sleep deprivation in normal-weight young individuals. *Molecular Metabolism* 2016;5(12):1175-86.

Chapter 10

51   Practice guideline update summary: Mild cognitive impairment. Report of the Guideline Development, Dissemination, and Implementation Subcommittee of the American Academy of Neurology. *Neurology* 2018;90:1-10.

52   Nagamatsu LS, Handy T, Hsu L, et al. Resistance training promotes cognitive and functional brain plasticity in seniors with probable mild cognitive impairment. *Arch Intern Med* 2012;172(8):666-668.

53   Suzuki T, Shimada H, Makizako H, et al. A randomized controlled trial of multicomponent exercise in older adults with mild cognitive impairment. *PLOS ONE* 2013;8(4):e61483.

54   Braiding involves moving sideways while crossing one foot in front of the other, stepping through, and then crossing that foot behind the other, and stepping through again.

Chapter 11

55   Waye A, Trudeau VL. Neuroendocrine disruption: more than hormones are upset. *J Toxicol Environ Health B Brit Rev* 2011;14(5-7):270-291.

56   Hadjivassiliou M, Grunewald RA, Davies-Jones GAB. Gluten sensitivity as a neurological illness. *Journal of Neurology, Neurosurgery & Psychiatry* 2002;72:560-563.

57   Rris A, Leblanc S. Maternal and fetal exposure to pesticides associated to genetically modified foods in Eastern Townships of Quebec, Canada. *Reproductive Toxicology* 2011;31(4):528-33.

Chapter 12

58   https://www.apa.org/news/press/releases/stress/2016/coping-with-change.pdf

59   http://www.nydailynews.com/news/national/stress-levels-soar-america-30-30-years-article-1.1096918

60 Klugman R. Stress: *The Nature and History of Engineered Grief.* Greenwood Publishing Group, 1992, p. 15.

61 Selye H. A syndrome produced by diverse nocuous agents. *Nature* 1936; 138(3479):32. The monograph can be viewed here: http://bit.ly/2HnTcHk

62 McEwen BS, Morrison JH. Brain on Stress: vulnerability and plasticity of the prefrontal cortex over the life course. *Neuron* 2013;79(1):16-29.

63 Hozel BK, Carmody J, Vangel M. Mindfulness practice leads to increases in regional brain matter density. *Psychiatry Res* 2011;191(1)36-43.

64 Hozel BK, Carmody J, Evans KC. Stress reduction correlates with structural changes in the amygdala. *Social Cogn Affect Neurosci* 2010;5(1)11-17.

Chapter 13

65 Buettner, D. Lessons for Living Longer from the People Who've Lived the Longest. National Geographic Press, 2010.

66 Simopolos AP. The importance of the ratio of omega-6/omega-3 essential fatty acids. *Biomed Pharmacother* 2002;56(8):365-79.

67 Hoojimans CR, Pasker-de Jong PC, de Vries RB, et al. The effects of long-term omega-3 supplementation on cognition and Alzheimer's pathology in animal models of Alzheimer's disease: a systematic review and meta-analysis. *J Alzheimers Dis* 2012;28(1):191-209.

68 Albert BB, Derraik JGB, Cameron-Smith D, et al. Fish oil supplements in New Zealand are highly oxidised and do not meet label content of n-3 PUFA. *Scientific Reports* 2015;5:Article number 7928.

69 Forrest KY, Stuhldreher WL. Prevalence and correlates of vitamin D deficiency in US adults. *Nutr Res* 2011;31(1):48-54.

70 Landel V, Annweiler C, Millet P. Vitamin D, cognition and Alzheimer's disease: the therapeutic benefit is in the D-tails. *J Alzheimer's Dis* 2016;53(2):419-444.

71 Sotirchos ES, Bhargava P, Eckstein C, et al. Safety and immunologic effects of high-vs low dose cholecalciferol in multiple sclerosis. *Neurology* 2016;86:1-9.

72 World Health Organization. The World Health Report, 2002: Reducing risks, promoting healthy life. Geneva, Switzerland.

73 Wessells KR, Singh GM, Brown KH. Estimating the global prevalence of inadequate zinc intake from national food balance sheets: effects of methodological assumptions. *PLOS ONE* 2012:7(11) ;e50565.

74 Ervin RB, Kennedy-Stephenson J. Mineral intakes of elderly adult supplement and non-supplement users in the third national health and nutrition examination survey. *J Nutr.* 2002:132(11):3422-7.

75 Malavolta M, Piacenza F, Basso A, et al. Serum copper to zinc ratio: relationship with aging and health status. *Mechanisms of Aging and Development* 2015;151:93-100.

76 Blanke ML VanDongen AMJ. Activation mechanisms of the NMDA receptor, Chapter 13. *Biology of the NMDA receptor*, Van Dongen AM (editor), CRC Press/Taylor & Francis; Boca Raton, FL, 2009.

77 Rosanoff A, Weaver CM, Rude RK. Suboptimal magnesium status in the United States: are the health consequences underestimated? *Nutr Rev* 2012;70(3):153-64.

78 Lazarus B, Chen Y, Wilson FP, et al. Proton pump inhibitor use and risk of chronic kidney disease. *JAMA Intern Med* 2016;176(2):238-46.

79 Gomm W, von Holt K, Thome F. Association of proton pump inhibitors with risk of dementia: a pharmacoepidemiological clams data analysis. *JAMA Neurol* 2016;73(4):410-416.

80 Shealy, C.N., (November 2005). Transdermal absorption of magnesium. (Abstract) 99th Annual Scientific Assembly of the Southern Medical Association, page S18.

81 Lonning PE, Berge EO, Bjornslett M, et al. White blood cell BRCA1 promoter methylation status and ovarian cancer risk. *Ann Intern Med* 2018. [Epub ahead of print 16 January 2018] doi: 10.7326/M17-0101.

82 Ravaglia G, Forti P, Maioli F, et al. Homocysteine and folate as risk factors for dementia and Alzheimer's disease. *Am J Clin Nutr* 2005;82(3):636-43.

83 Morris MC, Wany Y, Barnes LL, et al. Nutrients and bioactives in green leafy vegetables and cognitive decline. *Neurology* 2017. Published ahead of print.

84 Turner RS, Thomas RG, Craft S, et al. A randomized double-blind, placebo-controlled trial of resveratrol for Alzheimer's disease. *Neurology* 2015;85(16):1383-1391.

85 Sehgal N, Gupta A, Valli RK, et al. Withania somnifera reverses Alzheimer's disease pathology by enhancing low-density lipoprotein receptor-related protein in liver. *Proc Natl Acad Sci USA* 2012;109(9):3510-3515.

86 Lai PL, Naidu M, Sabaratnam V. Neurotrophic properties of the Lion's mane medicinal mushroom, Hericium erinaceus (Higher Basidiomycetes) from Malaysia. *Int J Med Mushrooms* 2013;15(6):639-54.

87 Zhang J, An S, Hu W, et al. The neuroprotective properties of Hericium erinaceus in glutamate-damaged differentiated PC12 cells and an Alzheimer's disease mouse model. *Int J Mol Sci* 2016;17(11):1810.

88 Krahl SE, Clark KB. Vagus nerve stimulation for epilepsy: a review of central mechanisms. Surg Neurol Int 2012;3(suppl 4):S255-259.

89 Vonck K, Boon P. The mechanism of action of vagus nerve stimulation therapy. *European Neurological Review* 2008;3(2):97-100.

90 Zobel A, Joe A, Freymann N, et al. Changes in regional cerebral blood flow by therapeutic vagus nerve stimulation in depression: an exploratory approach. *Psychiatry Research* 2005;139(3)165-179.

91 Pardo JV, Sheikh SA, Schwindt GC, et al. Chronic vagus nerve stimulation for treatment-resistant depression decreases resting ventromedial prefrontal glucose metabolism. *Neuroimage* 2008;42(2):879-889.

92 Iaccarino HF, Singer AC, Martoell AJ, et al. Gamma frequency entrainment attenuates amyloid load and modifies microglia. *Nature* 2017;540:230-235.

93 *Photobiomodulation for improving brain function in dementia* (PBM Dementia), University of California, San Francisco. ClinialTrials.gov identifier: NTC03160027.

94 Saltmarche AE, Naesser MA, Ho KF. Significant improvement in cognition in mild to moderately severe dementia cases treated with transcranial plus intranasal photomodulation: case series report. *Photomed Laser Surg* 2017;35(8):432-441.

95 Technischer Uberwachungsverein

96 Oster G. Auditory beats in the brain. *Scientific American* 1973;229(4).

97 Bliss TVP, Cooke SF. Long-term potentiation and long-term depression: a clinical perspective. *Clinics* 2011;66(S1):3-17.

98 Jackson MP, Rahman A, Lafon B, et al. Animal models of transcranial direct current stimulation: methods and mechanisms. *Clin Neurophysiol* 2016;127(11):3425-3454.

99 Leuchter AF, Cook IA, Jin Y, et al. The relationship between brain oscillatory activity and therapeutic effectiveness of transcranial magnetic stimulation in the treatment of major depressive disorder. *Front Hum Neurosci* 2013;7:37.

100 Stagg CJ, Best JG, Stephenson MC, et al. Polarity-sensitive modulation of cortical neurotransmitters by transcranial stimulation. *J Neurosci* 2009;29(16):5202-6.

101 Liss S, Liss B. Physiological and therapeutic effects of high frequency electrical pulses. *Integr Physiol Behavioral Sci* 1996;31(2):88-94.

102   Bai W, Liu T, Dou M, et al. Repetitive transcranial magnetic stimulation reverses AB1-42-induced dysfunction in gamma oscillation during working memory. *Curr Alzheimer Res* 2018; Jan 9. doi: 10.2174/1567205015666180110114050. [Epub ahead of print]

103   Southworth S. A study of the effects of cranial electrical stimulation on attention and concentration. *Integr Physiol Behav Sci* 1999;34(1):43-53.

104   Smith RB. Cranial electrotherapy stimulation in the treatment of stress related cognitive dysfunction, with an 18 month follow up. *Journal of Cognitive Rehabilitation* 1999;17(6):14-18.

105   Brown RP, Gerberg PL. Non-drug treatments for ADHD: New options for kids, adults, and clinicians. *Integr Physiol Behav Sci* 1999;34(1):43-53.

Epilogue

106   Lacey RE, Kumari M, Bartley M. Social isolation in childhood and adult inflammation: Evidence from the National Child Development Study. *Psychoneuroimmunology* 2014;50:85-94.

107   Shao Y, Yan G, Xuan Y, et al. Chronic social isolation decreases glutamate and glutamine levels and induces oxidative stress in the rat hippocampus. *Behav Brain Res* 2015;282:201-208.

108   Yuan L, Liu S, Bai X, et al. Oxytocin inhibits lipopolysaccharide-induced inflammation in microglial cells and attenuates microglial activation in lipopolysaccharide-treated mice. *J Neuroinflammation* 2016;13:77.

109   Gutkowska J, Jankowski M, Antunes-Rodrigues J. The role of oxytocin in cardiovascular regulation. *Braz J Med Biol Res* 2014;47(3):206-214.

INDEX

Printed in Great Britain
by Amazon